Life Events and Emotional Disorder Revisited

Life Events and Emotional Disorder Revisited explores the variety of events that can occur, their inherent characteristics and how they affect our lives and emotions, and in turn their impact on our mental health and wellbeing.

The book focuses on current social problems nationally and internationally, showing the reach of life events research including those linked to Covid-19. It also discusses trauma experiences and how they fit in the life events scheme. To underpin the various life event dimensions identified (such as loss, danger and humiliation), the authors have developed an underlying model of human needs, jeopardised by the most damaging life events. This includes attachment, security, identity and achievement. The book brings together classic research findings with new advances in the field of life events research, culminating in a new theoretical framework of life events, including new discussions on trauma, on positive events and an online methodology for measuring them. Additionally, it draws out the clinical implications to apply the research for improved practice.

The book will be of interest to researchers, clinicians and students in psychology, psychiatry and psychotherapy in broadening their understanding of how life events impact on individuals and how this can be applied to enhance clinical practice and stimulate future research.

Antonia Bifulco is Professor and Director at the Centre for Abuse and Trauma Studies at Middlesex University. She began her career as part of the original Brown & Harris team who developed their novel approach to life events methodology. She is a psychologist with expertise in lifetime development, trauma, attachment and emotional disorder.

Ruth Spence is a Post-Doctoral Research Fellow at the Centre of Abuse and Trauma Studies at Middlesex University. She undertook her PhD at the University of Cambridge and is expert in forensic and clinical issues and mental health in young people.

Lisa Kagan is a Research Fellow at the Centre for Abuse and Trauma Studies at Middlesex University. Her interests include investigating risks for clinical disorder in youth and adults and qualitative methods to explore the meaning of experience. She is also a Chartered Clinical Psychologist working in IAPT services.

Life Events and Emotional Disorder Revisited

Research and Clinical Applications

Antonia Bifulco,
Ruth Spence, and Lisa Kagan

Routledge
Taylor & Francis Group

LONDON AND NEW YORK

First published 2021
by Routledge
2 Park Square, Milton Park, Abingdon, Oxon OX14 4RN

and by Routledge
52 Vanderbilt Avenue, New York, NY 10017

Routledge is an imprint of the Taylor & Francis Group, an informa business

British Library Cataloguing-in-Publication Data
A catalogue record for this book is available from the British Library

Library of Congress Cataloging-in-Publication Data
A catalog record has been requested for this book

ISBN: 978-0-367-37157-9 (hbk)
ISBN: 978-0-367-37158-6 (pbk)
ISBN: 978-0-429-35290-4 (ebk)

Typeset in Baskerville
by codeMantra

To all researchers who use their minds and methods to understand the world, for social good.

To our families who sustain us.

Contents

Figures

Tables

Foreword

This book contains a wealth of information about wide-ranging aspects of emotional disorder, aetiological, methodological and clinical. But it also has practical implications: that investigator-based measures – which can ensure greater comparability in assessment between cases with such disorder and control participants without it – are more likely to further understanding than respondent-based ones. The latter include checklist and simple questionnaires, where data may not be strictly comparable due to the respondents' differing interpretations of the wordings such as "serious illness" or "excess noise at work". However, hitherto most investigator-based measures have involved face-to-face interviews where the interviewer has been trained to ask relevant additional probes in order to establish ratings with this kind of high inter-rater reliability. But interviews are costly and time-consuming with the consequence that investigator-based measures are less often used than the various questionnaire measures available. In order to address this issue, the authors of this volume are introducing a new computerised version of one of the earlier investigator-based interviews, the LEDS (Life Events and Difficulties Schedule), in the hope that it will bypass the need for the expensive interview. They introduce us to the CLEAR (Computerised Life Events Assessment Record) which they have recently been developing for this purpose. Such a message makes this publication very timely at the start of this new decade.

In its first decade, the LEDS was developed to explore the onset of schizophrenic psychosis episodes by George Brown and Jim Birley at London's Institute of Psychiatry. They were concerned to maximise inter-rater reliability in rating life events occurring in the immediate pre-onset period, so they focused on what "counted" as an event and on its "independence" (whether it had come from outside or had occurred as a result of something to do with the participant such as their argumentativeness, neglect or simple decision to act in a particular way). This procedure involved much deliberation that was then manualised: it is rumoured that George and Jim once spent a whole afternoon discussing whether it should count as an event when a patient reported the eye of his goldfish had fallen out and floated round the bowl for hours a few days before his episode. The rules subsequently embodied that it should not count as a LEDS event as there seemed to be no consequences of substance for that patient and his life beyond the macabre, almost surreal, image of a disembodied eye seeming to follow the participant's every move. Furthermore, had it even happened or was it a prodromal hallucination? Later, systematisation of the guidelines for including incidents as events followed similar procedures of debate and decision by consensus of the research team (four or more researchers). In the case of pet experiences, the LEDS earned a reputation for pro-mammal discrimination: incidents concerning birds, fish and reptiles hardly ever counted, while those involving dogs, cats and ponies – even a reindeer – were not infrequent.

In its second decade, during which I joined George's team now at London University's Bedford College, the LEDS focused on clinical depression both among patients and in a representative community sample. Certain key rating distinctions were established between short- and long-term negative implications and between contextual and reported threatfulness with the final evolution of the rating of "severe event" later used in so many studies. It became clear how often events which were the most compelling had no easy description in a checklist for they involved secrets, lies or deceptions; though it was only later that we came to understand that not being believed after disclosing a long-held secret was just as devastating as a revelation (learning of another's secret, e.g. that the woman you had thought was your older sister was really your mother). In this second phase, the measure was also pioneered in the Outer Hebrides where George was able to use his anthropology training to add extensions about intercultural use of the instrument to the growing LEDS manuals.

The next phase when Antonia joined the team was perhaps its most creative, developing qualitative characteristic dimensions of events such as loss, danger, humiliation, intrusiveness, commitment, fresh start, anchoring and goal-frustration; it also saw the formulation of new instruments outside the LEDS, measures of coping strategies, self-evaluation and childhood experience of care and abuse. The MacArthur Foundation financed an update of the schedules and manuals for use in a special LEDS training week in Pittsburgh in 1989 where Antonia played a pivotal role.

In the decades since then, the instrument has seen consolidation rather than new development. Many researchers have been trained and have used the instrument to look at emotional disorder in their own chosen populations so the rating rules for different cultures such as Zimbabwe, Pakistan and subgroups of immigrants in the UK and Canada were amplified. A few new qualitative characteristic dimensions were elaborated by researchers outside the team exploring different disorders, for example, "conflict over speaking out" in functional dysphonia samples, "pudicity" among restricting anorexia patients and "escape" in those with conversion disorder. But, as this book attests, in the uncertainty prevailing among those involved in gene-environment (GXE) interaction analysis of major depression and the serotonin transporter length polymorphism, very few have sought to re-examine with more investigator-based measures. This volume is thus especially timely.

But what makes this book particularly welcome now is that 2020 sees the world in a pandemic where computerised socialisation has become a source of emotional rescue. Many now have become familiar with typing, websites, Skype and Zoom and do not worry about disclosing feelings of vulnerability and joy online. Moreover, many now have mobile phones which give easy access to the internet. In parallel, IT programmes have evolved to an extent which makes the detailed extensions needed by CLEAR more feasible to achieve.

One of the aspects of the LEDS which these authors applaud is its attention to time order. This is also crucial in relation to whatever dependent variable is being examined, whether disorder or wellbeing: events following after onset logically cannot be considered of aetiological relevance. Somehow, someone has got to let the computer know a date of "onset" to compare with the inputted dates of the events. It is not obvious exactly how CLEAR dealt with this in the studies reported here, but with time and effort, the programme should easily be developed to accommodate this issue. There are other issues concerning the dependent variable which may require consideration in this context. The authors do not elaborate here on the topic of differentiating major depression from minor depression, although it was an area which initially delayed acceptance of Brown's team's work. The intervening decades have seen such detailed work on successive DSM and ICD definitions that the issue is less pressing in 2020, but research with other disorders may find itself facing parallel issues. Nor do the volume's authors drag readers through the debates about categorical versus dimensional measures of disorder (caseness of depression yes/no? vs symptom score) with their resulting different implications for multivariate statistical analysis. I once – paradoxically – had the greatest fun in finding that you could achieve the opposite answer to the question "Is there interaction between provoking agent and vulnerability factor" using exactly the same data set, and exactly the same cut-offs for the independent variables, but according to whether it was a categorical measure of clinical depression based on the PSE (Present Sate Examination) interview or a dimensional one (PSE-score; see Brown, Harris & Lemyre, 1991). But there is more to such issues of the dependent variable than mere sport. As the authors of this book outline, the millennium saw the dawning of another quest for another interaction to explain depression – a gene-environment one, where the serotonin transporter length polymorphism is hypothesised to interact with one or more of the environmental factors detailed here; and where the indications so far amount to "now you see it, now you don't". However, it seems possible that the key here may lie with the dependent variable, that the GXE effect might involve *chronic or recurring* depression, not simple experience of any one episode above the clinical threshold (Brown et al, 2013). This of course lurches the whole quest forward to search out perpetuating factors alongside provoking ones, something already begun in the 1990s (Brown & Moran, 1994; Brown, Harris, Hepworth & Robinson, 1994).

Some of the most promising practical implications of this volume are those involving therapeutic work: having online input from CLEAR could give a clinician valuable information as a background to session work. The patients could provide the relevant input in their own time and place, with permission to start and stop whenever they felt so compelled so long as it was available for the therapist in time, a blessed counteraction to user fatigue. As well as saving time, this might even sometimes provide an eye opener for the clinician. Again, the Covid-19 lockdown has meant that people with disorder are now more likely to consent to this, having become more used to having therapy online.

The onward journey to greater understanding and more effective treatment of depression is likely to be long and challenging, but this book marks an important step on the way.

Tirril Harris Institute of Psychiatry, Kings College London, May 2020

References

Brown, G.W., Ban, M., Craig, T.K., Harris, T.O., Herbert, J., & Uher, R. (2013). Serotonin transporter length polymorphism, childhood maltreatment, and chronic depression: A specific gene–environment interaction. *Depression and Anxiety, 30*(1), 5–13.

Brown, G.W., Harris, T.O., Hepworth, C., & Robinson, R. (1994). Clinical and psychosocial origins of chronic depressive episodes. II: A patient enquiry. *British Journal of Psychiatry, 165,* 457–465.

Brown, G.W., Harris, T.O., & Lemyre, L. (1991). Now you see it, now you don't - some considerations on multiple regression. In: D. Magnusson, L. R. Bergman, G. Rudinger, & B. Torestad (Eds.), *Problems and methods in longitudinal research: Stability and change* (pp. 67–94). Cambridge: Cambridge University Press.

Brown, G.W. & Moran, P. (1994). Clinical and psychosocial origins of chronic depressive episodes. I: A community survey. *British Journal of Psychiatry, 165,* 447–456.

Preface

The 'Bedford Square team' led by George Brown and Tirril Harris at Bedford College (later Royal Holloway), University of London, was acknowledged as a source of great creative research which gave insight into issues of how inequality can result in emotional disorder. Their focus on life events and stress in women hit the crest of the feminist movement in the 1970s, and the subsequent focus on vulnerability and childhood experience extended this with a life history focus in the 1980s and 1990s. Their method of accurately capturing experience through interview narrative of everyday lives fascinated a research audience raised on checklist questionnaires. It invited experts from various disciplines internationally to consider this new method of capturing the essence of adversity in narrative that could be quantified for statistical analysis in relation to depression. The Life Events and Difficulties Schedule (LEDS) was the first foray into capturing contextualised adversity experience in this way. Taking a modest time frame (12 months), it prompted narrative of recent life change through semi-structured interviews with Londoners and made the investigator, not respondents, responsible for scoring characteristics of experience. So, while the interviewers held the keys to the scoring and interpretation, it was the respondents who provided the rich life stories – a veritable treasure to be collected. It was a heady experience for the many young researchers who learned their research craft in the four decades of the teams' life in their Bloomsbury offices.

I joined the Brown and Harris team in the autumn of 1974 to take up an ESRC-funded PhD on the topic of loss of mother in childhood and adult depression. Exploring this vulnerability model turned into *my* life course exploration of risk factors for depression. George Brown was my supervisor and Tirril Harris my day-to-day guide on becoming a researcher. I worked with the team managing some projects and heading others until the year 2000 when the MRC funding ended for this brand of social research and the new genetic era was underway. In retirement, Brown and Harris moved to Kings College London. I remained with the research team at Royal Holloway, still located in Bedford Square London to complete the MRC data analysis, to publish and to work on translating the research into practice. This has continued through the Centre for Abuse and Trauma Studies (CATS), now at Middlesex University.

The rich information produced over the decades held true to its promise and has furnished a wealth of publishable data right up to the current day. The principles around measurement remain unchanged – but these have often been compromised or forgotten in our lean research times. The maxim – the more you put in, the more you get out – still holds true. Whilst much in modern research into depression has expanded its scope (to include, e.g. biological investigation along with that psychological and sociological) and improved analysis techniques (statistical modelling to allow for ever greater sophistication) in illuminating underlying mechanisms for disorder, the semi-structured interviews and subtle rating schemes initiated by the Bedford Square team under Brown's leadership have rarely been improved upon. Of course, there was much that was difficult and would have been made swifter with our modern technology – painstaking relistening to interviews and selective transcription for scoring – consensus meetings to ensure reliability – centralised data analysis reliant on key programmers. These issues made the work painstaking and relatively slow to produce. But the bright theoretical insights and rich analysis produced were clearly worth the effort. The approach was in large part inductive – it took its lessons from the respondents, not the professionals, in producing realistic models of individuals coping, or failing to cope, in hostile or socially deprived environments. It produced a bank of extraordinary life interviews still vibrant and relevant to today's challenges around relationships, material hardships and traumatic early lives.

This book attempts to keep that spirit alive whilst making concessions to modern ways of working. It seeks to blend the old knowledge with the new. It revisits the team's research findings back to the 1970s and synthesises them with updates from the present day. No doubt, there will be both too little detail, or too much, for some readers. It is a fine line to tread in reviewing decades of studies. Some of the rating schemes described even I find a little labyrinthine looking back – we have simplified descriptions of measures and findings to keep the reader engaged. As members of the CATS research team working at Middlesex University, we have extended the earlier published work in various ways. For example, we focus on new and current social problems nationally and internationally in showing the reach of life events research, we focus on trauma experiences and how they fit in the life event scheme, we have further developed the positive events research to look at wellbeing and we introduce a new online application of the LEDS interview, named CLEAR (Computerised Life Event Assessment Record). To underpin the various iterations of life event dimensions, we have speculated on a new underlying model of human needs which indicates how these are jeopardised by the most damaging life events. Thus, a focus on attachment, security, identity and achievement. This latter is new and speculative but aims to explicate further what we mean by a severe life event and how it can be damaging to an individual. How the outer world affects the inner psychological world. In this, we hope we have honoured the original research and respected the many, many hours of respondent time generously given to the work over the years.

Antonia Bifulco,
CATS, Middlesex University
May 2020

Acknowledgements

There are a great many individuals who make up a research team and who have contributed to research in programme grant outputs mentioned here. In addition to George Brown who was Principle Investigator of the MRC-programme grants up to the year 2000, working closely with Tirril Harris, we recognise the substantial input from Patricia Moran, Berenice Andrews, James Nazroo and Angela Edwards in the life event research and our longer-term colleagues Catherine Jacobs and Amanda Bunn who worked in the original team and still work with us. In addition, we appreciate the input of Tom Craig who aided with the psychiatric evaluations and Laurence Letchford who oversaw the computer analysis. We also acknowledge the substantial contribution of Helen Fisher, Georgina Hosang, Stephen Nunn and Mike Smith to the CLEAR project, designing and testing the online measure of life events. We are also very grateful for the editing work on this book undertaken by Amanda Bunn and Helen Fisher as well as to Tirril for writing the Foreword.

Of course, our greatest debt is to the many individuals who took part in our research, spending hours telling us their life stories, sharing very intimate experiences with great generosity, on the understanding that this would help others in the future. We hope we have fulfilled this expectation.

A note on the research team

'The Bedford Square team' refers to researchers on the MRC-research programmes for which George Brown was Principle Investigator from 1977 to 1999. In this, he was aided by Tirirl Harris with the final programme transferred to Antonia Bifulco following George Brown's retirement. The programme of research was initially at Bedford College which merged with Royal Holloway, University of London in the 1980s, with the research team located in Bloomsbury, first with offices in Harley St/New Cavendish St and later in Bedford Square, London. The research team was originally known as the Social Research team (Bedford College), then the Socio-Medical Research Centre (Royal Holloway), but often also termed the Bedford Square team after the college and location. Post George Brown's retirement and move to Kings College London to focus on biological aspects of vulnerability as well as interventions, the data analysis and publication were continued by Antonia and colleagues at Royal Holloway as the Lifespan Research Group and latterly at Middlesex University as the Centre for Abuse and Trauma studies, where the authors are currently located. Training on the different research interviews described now occurs at CATS[1] under the lifespan training label.[2]

The research projects conducted by the Bedford Square team were in the main conducted in the London community with the use of general practice lists for selecting respondents. Those whose findings are specifically referred to in this book are listed in Appendix 1. The measures utilised and key papers for sample description are also listed.

Examples provided in the text are all taken from research interviews undertaken by the team. Consistent with the ethical agreement, they are identified by a fictitious first name to preserve anonymity. Occasionally, other elements such as location, names of others or work role are changed to make sure these are unidentifiable. However, all the key contextual aspects are kept as in the original interview. In all projects, ethical permission was provided by the university involved and the relevant health ethical board. Informed and signed consent was obtained from all participants.

Notes

1 https://catsresearch.org.uk/
2 https://lifespantraining.org.uk/

1   Introduction

Adversity is always around us. It has important impacts on our lives, our state of mind and our wellbeing. When we experience life events, the change to our personal circumstances requires adaptation and coping. Such change can at times be minor or even positive, but when the events are both significant and negative, the impacts can be overwhelming. These events can threaten and damage our relationships, roles or material possessions with implications for our future lives. This can challenge our safety, close attachments or sense of identity or cherished achievements. For example, many severe life events involve loss. Amongst the worst is the death of people close to us. This will usually leave us bereft, affecting not only our mood but also our daily roles and routines and our ability to look forward to the future. It requires a period of mourning to process and accept the loss, and to find a way to renew investment in our roles and other relationships (Murray-Parkes, 1988). It often leads to depression as our basic attachment system is threatened. Many people are unaware that a similar process is needed to cope with other negative life events involving loss, such as losing a home or a job or a friendship. All require substantial adaptation and have implications for mental health. We hope to show in this book that problems with mental health, particularly around emotional disorder such as depression and anxiety, are in a large part due to the adverse things that happen to us. We aim to explore how life events can damage us emotionally.

Some losses may be related to conflict events which also invoke danger. For example, partner separation involving loss can sometimes follow a period of intense argument or violence which has danger elements. Coping is required both with the conflict and then with the loss. The challenges around coping with conflict involve dealing with danger and resulting vigilance, to which our instinct may be of flight or fight, or indeed, to hide. These events affect our sense of security – the world may seem suddenly unsafe and unsure. Disappointments too, such as failing an exam or a key job interview after hope of a new career direction, can lead to feelings that our life plans are de-railing and our achievement plans extinguished. Most of us think of life events around the life categories involved (e.g. 'education' or 'partner' or 'housing'). But identifying experiences of loss, danger and disappointment under the heading of 'severe' life event is a different and effective way of explaining how adverse changes in our daily lives, across various categories, impinge on us personally and psychologically. Thus, we learn how such events can undermine our feelings of being safe, being close to others, being a worthy person or being successful. These threats can provide important indicators for how emotional damage occurs as well as how interventions should be focused. When we encounter severe events involving loss or danger, the likelihood of triggering a clinical depression or anxiety state is greatly increased (Brown & Harris, 1978). Exploring the variety of events that can occur, their inherent characteristics and how they affect our lives and emotions is the focus of this book.

It now seems intuitive that negative life events bring about depression, but for greater precision, the mechanisms involved, the identification of the types of events most harmful and the types of people most affected has involved decades of study. The study of life events has a long and multi-disciplinary history in relation to health. It can be traced from medicine and psychiatry, through psychoanalysis and psychology, to sociology and epidemiology. Its multi-disciplinary range fits with the modern notion of the integrated bio-psycho-social model of the causes of clinical disorder. For example, early in the 20th century, Freud's writings on *Mourning and Melancholia* (Freud, 1924) explained the linkages between bereavement and depression. He considered two different processes – in mourning, a person deals with the grief of losing a specific person or 'love object', this process taking place in the conscious mind and leading to resolution. Whereas in melancholia (or depression), a person grieves for a loss they are unable to fully comprehend or identify, the process taking place in the unconscious mind and remaining unresolved. Thus, Freud considered mourning to be a healthy and natural process of grieving a loss, while melancholia occurred when this turned towards psychopathology and disorder. This has parallels for positive and negative coping with a wider range of loss events.

Whilst modern interpretations of bereavement may differ, it is well established that some individuals can come through the stages of mourning without experiencing a clinical depression, whilst for others, the loss is unbearable and unresolvable. For Murray-Parkes, grief occurs in phases and takes into account our own history, experiences and the relationship with the deceased (Murray-Parkes, 1985). These factors can affect the mourning process. He identifies four stages of mourning which include feelings of shock or numbness, yearning and searching, disorganisation and despair, and finally recovery and reorganisation – the latter indicating a completed and healthy mourning process. Earlier experiences of loss in childhood, he argues, can affect whether individuals adapt to recent loss – the event can awaken echoes of prior losses which may not have been resolved, thus creating a vulnerability for future loss. This approach was much influenced by John Bowlby's attachment theory and the response of a child to losing a parent with emotions of fear, anger, frustration or grief (Bowlby, 1979), emotions carried through to adult life and affecting future relationships. These approaches focus on the psychological pain of losing someone close and how individuals have different capacities for coping based on early life experience. It lays a foundation for understanding not only the impact of severe loss events but also the factors which make some individuals more vulnerable. These will both be explored in this book.

Timing of severe life events in relation to emotional disorder is key. In order to show a causal effect, the event must come before the onset of disorder, but also relatively close in time if it is to have a casual role as a provoking agent. Yet people frequently experience a number of events, some more threatening than others, so determining a calendar of events that have happened in the recent period allows for scrutiny of which event is most likely to have brought about the disorder. Most individuals are aware of the event that has upset them most and led to overwhelming emotion and feelings of being helpless. But, sometimes, a significant event is not fully processed and remains a hidden provoking agent (Bifulco & Brown, 1996). This can be because events can happen in a sequence as a scenario unfolds and determining which is the most damaging point in that unfolding crisis can be unclear. (For instance, which was more painful – the angry rejecting row with a partner, his disclosure of infidelity, his leaving the home, or initiating divorce proceedings, all over a three-month period?) The important search for such sequences and timing of life events actually began in the 1950s, when the psychiatrist Adolf Meyer, having listened to his patients' narratives of different crises, investigated life events as a cause of clinical disorder. He developed a life chart system for recording the temporal relationships of these negative life experiences and depression from his careful observation of his patients' reported experience (Meyer, 1994). This was the first attempt to measure and chart life events systematically and was the precursor for the later intensive methods described in this book.

However, at some point thereafter, the timing of the event was disconnected from the life events with the innovation of brief checklist approaches in the 1960s (Holmes & Rahe, 1967). These only looked to the number of proscribed events experienced rather than their significance, sequence or timing in relation to disorder. It was left to the more sophisticated time-based interview approaches (Brown & Harris, 1978; Paykel, 1997) to investigate the events in full contextual scope as well as their timing and sequence. This then allowed for a focus on noting the particular event which preceded an onset of depression or anxiety to determine its characteristics in seeking mechanisms for psychological damage. Both methodological approaches (checklist questionnaires and in-depth interviews) have persisted in contemporary research and still constitute opposing theoretical and methodological viewpoints (Brown, 1993; Harkness & Monroe, 2016; McQuaid et al., 1992). It is only in recent times that online methods have bridged these two options (Bifulco, Spence, Nunn, Kagan et al., 2019).

Life events do not usually happen randomly to individuals. There are important social influences in bringing them about which are recognised in the social epidemiology of mental health. For example, early findings in the field of psychiatric epidemiology showed that rates of depression differed by location, even within cities, in relation to deprived areas – effectively 'postcode' distribution. A famous study in New York in the 1960s, The Midtown Manhattan Study, based on interviews of over a thousand individuals randomly selected, concluded that mental health risks were greatest among those with low socio-economic status

(SES) often grouped in key neighbourhoods (Kraines, 1964). This was to inform a generation of researchers who subsequently investigated depression amongst those disadvantaged, poor and socially excluded (Ross, 2000). However, it was through the investigation of severe life events occurring to individuals that the mechanisms of emotional damage from their adverse environment (whether domestic or neighbourhood) could be established.

George Brown and Tirril Harris were pioneers in this area and termed their seminal work on life events the 'Social Origins of Depression' in view of their recognition of social inequality and disadvantage as a key to common clinical disorder (Brown & Harris, 1978). In the mid-1970s, when they published, psychiatry was in the pendulum swing away from a biological view of clinical disorder and towards a social view, and their book was influential in showing a key role for social adversity through the experience of severe life events. Thus, they conducted community-based studies to show that the social environment can increase the likelihood of depression, particularly in poor city areas such as Camberwell in London, for those deprived and of lower social class, and groups with less power in society, for example, women. Their intensive study of the lives of inner-city London women highlighted ways in which hostile and impoverished environments can increase stress on individuals to the point where depressive disorder occurs.

Life events are not only the consequence of social adversity. Some of the disadvantage individuals' experience occurs earlier in life course development in relation to childhood, adolescent and early adult experience. This can also leave scarring (psychological, social and neurobiological) and can affect how individuals cope later in life. It may also lead to life events for example through difficulties in making close relationships which in turn results in relationship conflict or breakup events. It may also affect coping with such events in terms of helplessness or lack of emotional control. In the model described, these early life experiences are subsumed under vulnerability factors – those which make an individual more susceptible to both the occurrence and the impact of severe life events.

Brown and Harris' additional contribution was their innovative use of measurement. Their semi-structured interviews allowed individual respondents to openly narrate their recent stressful experience and, with interviewer use of probing questions, give detailed descriptions of the range of circumstances involved. This conveyed the full context which helped explain why the event was experienced as damaging and how it disrupted day-to-day lives. This methodology started a wave of interest in the accurate identification of severe life events and their prevalence by location and class – and the process by which these events could trigger clinical depression in individuals. This book seeks to describe the key methods and findings of this approach, and to update and extend these into later research for the benefit of students, researchers or those in clinical practice.

Community life events and trauma

Many life events are 'normative' and mark out life stages for an individual, and they are usually benign and can chart growth, advancement and achievement in stable circumstances. For example, starting higher education, getting married, the birth of children and starting retirement. However, these changes can be threatening or unpleasant under more unstable circumstances. For example, getting married can be problematic (e.g. if enforced or to an unsuitable, anti-social partner), and births can be problematic too for reasons of the mother's health, her poverty and poor housing or lack of a partner. Life events can also be non-normative in the sense of an unexpected disruption in the usual life course. These can come about because of conflict (e.g. domestic violence, mugging, sexual assaults, bullying) or through being badly let down or betrayed by close others (e.g. partner's infidelity, child's delinquency, parent's rejection). Other such events occur because of more widespread economic problems in the local community (e.g. redundancy, loss of benefits, homelessness).

However, life events can also have a basis in group and societal experience. Sometimes, this is on a very large scale for whole populations. Our most recent experience is through the Covid-19 pandemic (Brooks et al., 2020). Whilst largely unprecedented in recent times, it has affected every country and to greater or lesser extent every individual. For some, it is inconvenient but has not personally threatened their basic security – requiring, for example, social distancing, working from home, additional childcare responsibility. But for others, it has led to life-threatening illness, unexpected bereavement, reduced income, job loss or a dangerous work environment. All of these involve life events – many severe and many leading to longer-term difficulties. Managing the pandemic has created other negative conditions, which can inhibit coping and adaptation – for example, social distancing or shielding, limiting the visiting of those close to us who are sick and the giving and receiving of emotional support as well as curtailing cultural mourning practices at funerals or memorials. At the time of writing this book (May 2020), it is not known how or when the situation will resolve. Nor the extent of the impact on mental health nationally.

This current Covid-19 health crisis has brought to the public attention, epidemiologists who study the geographic patterning of illness and the spread of infectious disease. Epidemiological research is key to public health and to preventative medicine by tackling the study of populations and demography. There is a long and impressive history to such investigation, with much having had a London focus over many centuries. There is now resonance with the early origins of the discipline in the work of John Graunt in the mid-1600s who analysed the vital statistics of the citizens of London at a time of plague which killed thousands. In the year 1665 alone, a quarter of England's population died.[1] He developed a classification of death rates according to the causes of death, among which he included overpopulation. For example, he observed that the urban death rate exceeded the rural. He developed the life table which presented mortality in terms of survivorship – this leading to a statistical process still utilised not only for mortality but also for maintenance of therapeutic improvement (Kupfer et al., 1992). Two hundred years later, in the 1854 London cholera epidemic, similar principles were followed by physician John Snow, who traced the source of the outbreak to a particular water pump in Clerkenwell. He removed the pump handle thus reducing the death rate due to contaminated water. Snow's findings inspired fundamental changes in the water and waste systems of London, which led to similar changes in other cities, and a significant improvement in general public health around the world. As a result, not only mortality rates but also severe life events were reduced at societal levels with potential benefits to mental health.

Charles Booth, born in 1840, determined to study poverty and where it was located. He undertook a comprehensive scientific social survey of London life and developed his famous maps of poverty and inequality which mirrored health risk.[2] In modern times, we still talk of postcode risk in relation to deprivation and health access. Early interventions such as Sure Start actually utilised a postcode approach to identifying families at risk (Barnes et al., 2005). Yet as early as 1884, Booth found a quarter of the population of London lived in extreme poverty and produced maps of London, coloured street by street, to indicate the levels of poverty and wealth in 1888–1889. The influence of deprived locations on higher incidence of illness is thus long established. This has been applied to the study of life events as ways in which adversity impacts on individuals and this in turn to the prevalence of clinical disorder such as depression.

As well as contagious illnesses, toxic environmental influences can affect populations and at times differentially by poverty or location. This can include contaminated water (as in the John Snow example) but in modern times also radiation, for example, through catastrophic events such a radiation leakage from power plants (e.g. Chernobyl in the Ukraine or Fukushima Daiichi in Japan). The impacts on physical health are more direct (e.g. causing cancer) and have been charted by the World Health Organisation (WHO), but there are less visible health impacts such as on emotional stress, less often highlighted (Bennett, Repacholi, & Carr, 2006). The Chernobyl disaster can serve to illustrate the links between toxic environmental disasters and mental health. The disaster occurred on Saturday, 26 April 1986, at the No. 4 nuclear reactor in the Chernobyl Nuclear Power Plant, near the city of Pripyat in the north of the Ukrainian SSR.[3] The subsequent spread of radiation occurred geographically through wind currents and water, but also through effects on pasture and milk from cows. The main impacts were felt not only in Ukraine, but in neighbouring Belarus and Russia with some increases in cancer later found in Sweden and Poland in the following years up to 2005. Children aged under ten in neighbouring Belarus had striking increases in thyroid cancer and leukaemia peaking five to ten years after the explosion. However, there was a wider spread of other health consequences not resulting directly from the poisoning effects of radiation – that of anxiety and distress, increased smoking and alcohol use. These related to forced relocation, loss of home and jobs, and loss of life of family and friends as well as low access to health care in the resulting political turmoil. The recent powerful television series on Chernobyl also focused on the added failure of trust in the communist authorities, who in turn mistrusted scientific experts.[4] These are severe life events (including those involving trauma) on an international scale. A commentary on the WHO report states:

The Chernobyl accident led to extensive relocation of people, loss of economic stability, and long-term threats to health in current and possibly future generations. Widespread feelings of worry and confusion, as well as a lack of physical and emotional well-being were commonplace.... The accident has had a serious impact on mental health and well-being in the general population, mainly at a sub-clinical level that has not generally resulted in medically diagnosed disorders. Designation of the affected population as "victims" rather than "survivors" has led to feelings of helplessness and lack of control over their future. This has resulted in excessive health concerns or reckless behaviour, such as the overuse of alcohol and tobacco, or the consumption of mushrooms, berries and game from areas still designated as having high levels of radioactive caesium. https://allcountries.org/health/health_effects_of_the_chernobyl_accident_an_overview.html

Other such communal crises can come from extreme climatic impacts – such as tsunamis, floods or bushfires. Such catastrophic events can similarly lead to loss of housing and possessions, relocation and loss of life. Recent disturbing examples (in 2019) have included the Australian forest fires where 27 million acres of forest have caught ablaze and destroyed more than 2,000 houses in New South Wales, forcing thousands to seek shelter elsewhere.[5] Again, these circumstances create severe life events, including trauma for individuals, but on a national scale. Other international crises can be man-made through political conflict such as war where similarly whole populations are indiscriminately affected. This involves the additional fear of violence but also with enforced relocation with increased refugee and asylum-seeking travel, often under perilous circumstances. In modern times, this often involves dangerous journeys to the West from the Middle East or Africa where conflicts are rife. For those who cross the Mediterranean in dinghies, or who travel in sealed lorry containers to get refuge, this can lead to death.[5] But the journey and conditions requiring flight constitute severe life events, including trauma events and long-term difficulties for individuals and families involved. The refugees who survive are therefore at a particularly high risk of a range of clinical disorders (Heir, Blix, & Knatten, 2016; Horesh, Solomon, Zerach, & Ein-Dor, 2011).

The International Organization for Migration (IOM) states that 19,722 migrants had entered Europe by sea in 2017. Eighty per cent of the arrivals landed in Italy, with the rest coming to Spain and Greece. By then, around 154,416 migrants had arrived in Europe through the Mediterranean route in a year. In 2015, Syrians made up the largest contingent of refugees arriving in Italy, followed by Eritreans and people from the Horn of Africa. Since then, most refugees come from other African countries (Guinea, Nigeria, Ivory Coast, Gambia and Senegal) and Bangladesh. All these people suffer as a result. The IOM states:

Refugees arriving in Italy through Libya usually flee because of conflicts, persecution, poverty and reasons related to climate change. However, most of these migrants don't want to come to Europe. They travel to Libya, which is still perceived as a country where they can find a job and send money home, but the situation in Libya is very dangerous. Once they cross the borders, they become targets of abuse and human rights violations. They are kidnapped, detained illegally, tortured or raped and even killed. A majority of them don't want to come to Europe, but they see the sea crossing as the only way to save their lives.

https://www.dw.com/en/what-you-need-to-know-about-the-refugee-crisis-in-the-mediterranean-sea/a-38027330

However, even in normal life with no political conflict, or extreme climate events, individuals' lives can still involve varying rates and types of negative life events due to location or social deprivation. Whilst highest rates are often found in inner-city areas (with neighbourhood threats involving drugs, crime and violence or shortage of housing), rural events are also found in relation to unemployment, isolated housing, transport difficulties and flooding. Famers too are affected by both climate and animal health policies. When the BSE (Bovine Spongiform Encephalopathy) outbreak in cattle occurred in the UK in 2000, whilst there were some human losses attributed to the transmitted Creutzfeld-Jakob disease (CJD) illness, the largest human casualties proved to be suicides in farmers who had lost all their cattle and livelihoods, traumatised by burning the corpses of their cattle on huge pyres.[6] Other severe events were related to the closure of farms and need to travel for work from rural areas resulting in family separation, unemployment and financial hardship.

When Brown and Harris first examined rates of severe life events in Camberwell, an inner-city area of south London, they found that a third of individuals had experienced a severe life event in the prior 12 months. These severe events were more common in those working class as measured by main wage earners occupation. This also held for depression: whilst 15% of the sample were clinically depressed in the year, this was four times higher in those working class than those middle class (23% vs 6%) (Brown, 1972). Depression was also more common for those in certain life stages – it was disproportionately higher in women with children under age six living in the home. So, severe life events and depression were both more prevalent in those more socially disadvantaged females and in a relatively early adult life stage involved in childcare responsibilities.

Other researchers have similarly investigated such social inequalities in life event distribution and illness, in relation to occupation. The Whitehall Study (Stansfeld & Marmot, 1992) showed that of those employed in the civil service in the UK, the employees with least status in the organisation suffered the most severe life events and were most affected with both psychological and physical illness, including coronary heart disease. This included those working at lowest grades, for example, as messengers or doorkeepers who had a threefold higher rate of mortality than those who had the highest grades including administrators (Marmot, Shipley, & Rose, 1984). This sought to overturn the common view of midlife ill-health and privilege, for example, that heart attacks occurred through executive stress. Rather, it was among those with the least status and the least control over their lives who suffered the higher rates.

Such environmental explanations of life events can be understood in terms of Bronfenbrenner's model of socio-ecological development (Bronfenbrenner, 1995). Whilst his focus was on child development and the levels of influence from society, the model can be utilised to examine the many spheres of influence on the individual at a point in time from international or global, down to immediate family (see Figure 1.1). The model starts with the *microsystem* which includes the individual and their immediate environment such as with family, work, peers and the quality of these social systems. This is followed by the *mesosystem* which is the inter-relationship between the *microsystems*, for example, how a family communicates with the school and the impact that has on the child's behaviours. The *exosystem* follows, which reflects the relationship between settings in which the person may not play an active role in but nevertheless is affected, for example, the decisions made in a big company which affects a person's working hours which in turn impacts on their childcare setup. The *macrosystem* is the larger social and cultural context in which a person lives, and can impact on their lives through the effects of the nation's social and legal policy, and distribution of resources and services.

Thus, life events which are created in an international, national or neighbourhood setting are likely to be external to the individual and outside of their control, impacting on wider groups and communities. These can be viewed as 'independent' of the individual's own action in bringing them about. Enforced unemployment and financial difficulty due to a business going bankrupt, homelessness due to lack of social housing and long waiting lists, mugging due to street crime in the area and illness epidemics are all considered independent events. These are events likely to affect groups or populations due to a common

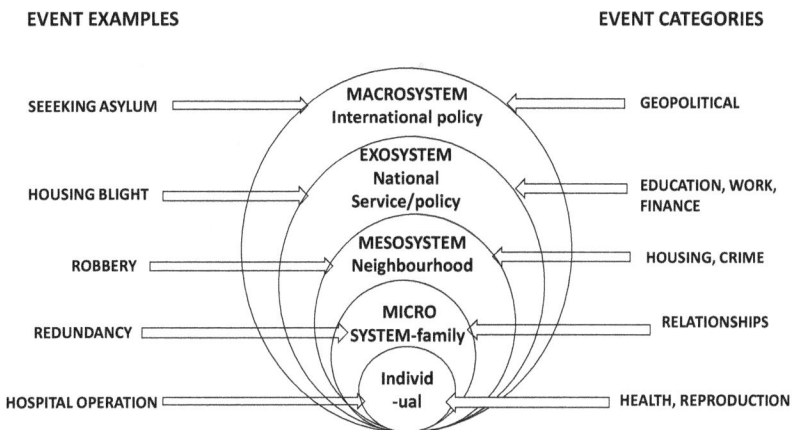

Figure 1.1 Socio-ecological approach to life events.

underlying circumstance. Such events can rise on a population basis given ongoing political conditions. Examples of how these types of events can map on to the socio-ecological social spheres are shown in Figure 1.1.

However, life events can sometimes occur as a consequence of the individual's own actions. For example, finalising a decision to leave a marriage, taking a new job and initiating a move to another city. These may improve life chances, reduce difficulties or maintain stability but may also set in train other adverse circumstances. Furthermore, other antisocial actions may initiate severe events for others, such as attacking a spouse, rejecting a child or defrauding an employer. These can be considered dependent upon the individual's own actions and volitions, even when understood in terms of other pressures and influences. The individual's psychological and life history contribution is likely to be greater for these types of events. This may involve personal vulnerability, personality influences or even earlier psychopathology such as personality disorder. This raises the issue of how vulnerability to emotional disorder can generate severe life events for others as well as making individuals more sensitised to the impact of severe events they experience. The next section will therefore outline the importance of vulnerability in relation to provoking agents and depression.

Vulnerability

Vulnerability involves the longer-term characteristics making an individual *susceptible* to the impact of severe life events (see Chapter 4 for a longer discussion). It can also increase an individual's risk of *experiencing* more severe life events – through perpetuation of adverse circumstances such as living in poor neighbourhoods or having a series of problematic relationships. Thus, it can invoke double jeopardy – greater experience of hardship and higher personal susceptibility in terms of clinical disorder. Both types emanate from similar sources and have a lifespan scope, with childhood neglect or abuse and other early life adversity playing a causal role. It also encompasses adversity in earlier adult life, particularly when prolonged over time, to show the accumulating ('dose') effects of multiple lifetime adversity on disorder for those who remain in disadvantaged circumstances (Bifulco, Bernazzani, Moran, & Ball, 2000; Dube et al., 2001). On the psychological front, it encompasses personal vulnerability, for example, through distorted attachment patterns involving mistrust and autonomy issues, leading to the generation of more relational events and greater sensitivity to such events. This in turn is associated with lower self-esteem and poorer crisis coping, and impaired emotional regulation in managing stress (Bifulco & Thomas, 2012).

Vulnerability is shown to work at social, psychological and biological levels. These are interrelated. For example, attachment theory provides an effective explanation of how a person's own early life maltreatment at the hands of parents, carers and can lead to enduring vulnerability (Bowlby, 1980). Patterns of secure, anxious or avoidant and disorganised interpersonal styles are identified which persist into adult life (Ainsworth, Blehar, Aters, & Wall, 1978; Main & Solomon, 1986). These can lead to enduring patterns of mistrust, for example, linked to fear of others, hostility to others and avoidance in relationships. It can also lead to anxious ambivalence with clinging behaviour in relationships through fear of abandonment. Bowlby viewed these behaviours emanating from childhood as persisting to adulthood through the mechanism of internal working models (or cognitive schema). This in turn has been linked to the individuals capacity to mentalise (understand one's own mind and that of others) and regulate emotions when under stress (Fonagy & Target, 1997). Individuals with distorted attachment patterns are more prone to recurrent emotional disorder and more vulnerable to the impact of severe life events (Bifulco, Moran, Ball, & Bernazzani, 2002). The linkages involve responses to early maltreatment, which itself has both a social and interpersonal basis and can lead to psychological developmental problems with cognitive distortions (low self-esteem, mistrust) and problem interpersonal behaviour (avoidance of closeness). When a severe life event occurs, particularly one in relationships, this trajectory can then lead to poorer coping (e.g. through self-blame or pessimism) and lack of crisis support due the unavailability of sustained close confiding relationships (Bifulco & Thomas, 2012). At this final point, depression or anxiety is highly likely to ensue. This shows the inter-play of social and psychological characteristics over time in creating risk for emotional disorder.

Biological influences are also involved. These are complex in that they can be directly linked to events through stress responses at the time of the event (see later GxE discussion of serotonin transporter gene and life events) or be linked through longer-term psychological vulnerability (such as insecure attachment style) or be a result of childhood experience which interacts with neurobiological or genetic factors to produce more or less sensitivity. These are all discussed in Chapter 4 on vulnerability and are briefly described here.

Genetic characteristics can be shown to interact *directly* with severe life events to cause clinical disorder and thus work as proximal vulnerability factors. The main line of investigation has been around low serotonin, an MOAO neurotransmitter which promotes low levels of norepinephrine responsible for features such as alertness and energy, attention, interest in life and motivation and reward, aspects depleted in depression (McCrory, De Brito, & Viding, 2010, 2012). Specifically, the serotonin transporter gene (5-HTT) is implicated in depression (Kendler, Kessler, Walters, MacLean, & et al., 1995). Studies in the last decade have found causal mechanisms involving interactions between the length polymorphism of the serotonin transporter gene (5-HTTPLR) and environmental adversity in the form of severe life events (Kim-Cohen et al., 2006).

In terms of biological links to *mediating* factors, such as attachment style, evidence has been presented around cortisol regulation and its role in tress response. Thus, insecure attachment style relates to dysregulated cortisol (Oskis, Loveday, Hucklebridge, Thorn, & Clow, 2010), a stress hormone known to become activated under threat and in relation to severe life events (Harris et al., 2000). Normally, this dissipates when the immediate danger is over, and coping is activated. But among individuals who have suffered chronic stress in childhood (e.g. through maltreatment), the mechanisms can become damaged with either a blocking or over-activation of cortisol reactivity. Individuals affected have greater hormonal response when life events occur which can hamper their coping capability.

There is also a '*differential susceptibility*' approach to genetic influences in response to adversity. This refers to sensitivity or hardiness characteristics of children and individuals related to childhood adversity and attachment characteristics which make some more sensitised to stressful experience (Bakermans-Kranenburg & IJzendoorn, 2007). The model states that individuals vary in their developmental plasticity and uses a flower analogy to illustrate that more plastic or malleable individuals ('orchids') are more susceptible than others who are hardier ('daisies') to environmental influences. The seven-repeat allele of the DRD4 gene has attracted particular attention, and children with this gene variant show more positive or negative outcomes with regard to behaviour problems and attachment security depending on the quality of maternal caregiving. However, the serotonin transporter, the 'short' 5-HTT promoter region allele, is also implicated. That is, children with this short-allele in their genetic makeup are more sensitised to both negative and supportive environments with either adverse or positive developmental sequelae to life events, so 'for better or for worse' (Belsky, Bakermans-Kranenburg, & Van IJzendoorn, 2007). Other explanations are sought in environmental stressors in the pre-natal environment which may result in pre-natal programming of developmental plasticity (Belsky & Pluess, 2009). Furthermore, alleles of certain dopamine, serotonin and monoamine oxidase genes appear to render individuals more susceptible to environmental influences and factors such as biological reactivity to stress and negative emotional reactivity also seem to make a contribution (Kennedy, 2013). Thus, research on neurobiological impacts illustrates how environmental factors impact on individual experiences and alter vulnerability to environmental influences (van IJzendoorn, Bakermans-Kranenburg, & Ebstein, 2011). Thus, neurobiological factors are argued to contribute to an individual's response to events and create greater sensitivity or resistance to negative events.

Vulnerability also has a major cognitive-affective component related to longer-term patterns of negative thinking and feeling which can work against coping with life events to manage adaptation and satisfy basic needs. For this, we invoke two models – Maslow's theory of need and Beck's theory of cognitive bias. The first explains people's needs in relation to psychological wellbeing, and how these might be challenged by severe life events to cause psychological disorder – for example, the need for safety or identity. The second explains why individuals might both catastrophise when crises occur and block positive coping through entrenched negative expectations of the world. Maslow's model displays need hierarchically, with food and shelter at the base and 'self-actualisation' at the peak (Maslow, 1971). In most cases, meeting the lower level needs is required, before the higher need ones can be fulfilled – thus, for example, the individual needs somewhere to live and food to eat, before investing time in additional education or creative achievement. We have formulated a new conceptual model which we will develop in this book to refer to the psychological needs challenged by severe life events. These we identify as needs for Attachment, Security, Identity and Achievement (ASIA), and all link to different theoretical psychological strands (e.g. attachment or self-identity or status hierarchy theories). These areas are differentially impacted when significant life events occur, and needs are newly exposed and unmet. Figure 1.2 shows Maslow's model onto which we have grafted these interpretative labels. We will refer to the ASIA model of need in more detail in following chapters.

Beck's negative cognitive triad has long been viewed as critical to understanding depression (Beck, 1967). This states that an individual can acquire negative cognitive biases or thought processes about the self, the world and the future, and these form underlying schemata derived from childhood which can then trigger further more intense negative views and expectations when severe life events occur. The corresponding cognitive response is of lowered self-esteem, increased fear of the outside world and increased pessimism. These characteristics all affect an individual's ability to cope and initiate positive action and access support. In Beck's triad, we prefer to subdivide his category of the 'world' to differentiate the relational or social and nonrelational environment. Thus, we have labelled a negative view of others (mistrust) as a fourth axis to link with the attachment theme to be developed. This also fits with the ASIA model and psychological needs (see Figure 1.3). We will later explore this model in relation to characteristics of severe life events such as loss, danger, humiliation and entrapment.

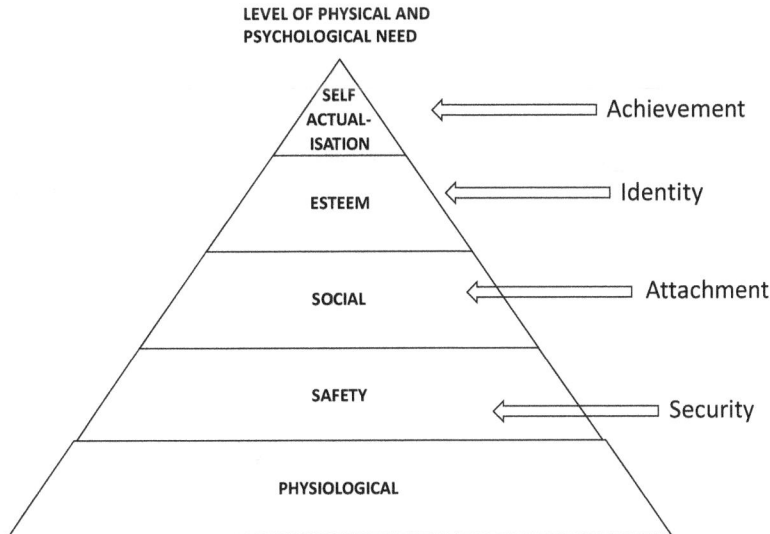

Figure 1.2 Maslow's hierarchy of needs and 'ASIA' categories.

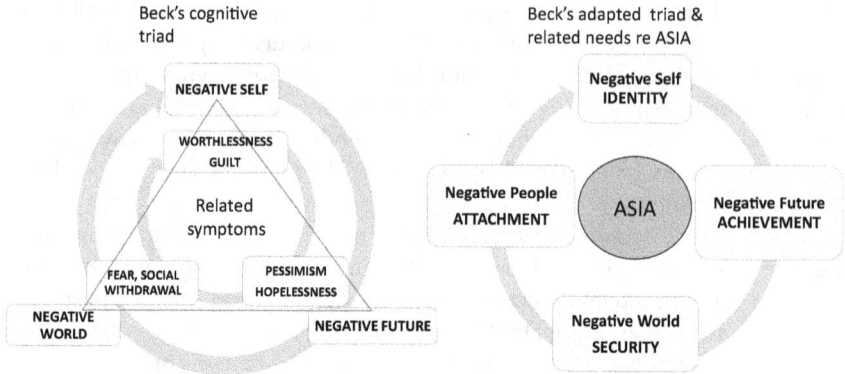

Figure 1.3 A model of negative cognitive schema and vulnerability.

Measuring life events

It is necessary to describe life events more fully by briefly introducing the Life Events and Difficulties Schedule (LEDS) as an interview measure since this will have a large focus in this book. (A more detailed account is provided in Chapter 2.) For those unfamiliar with the LEDS, it is a semi-structured face-to-face interview of about an hour which is audio-recorded and subsequently rated by the investigator on a number of scales according to predetermined manualised precedents. Life events are scored on a number of characteristics, including different *domains* ranging from health to education to interpersonal relationships. In addition, there are *categories* of events within these domains such as under education – starting school/university or taking exams. The *severity* rating is central – this comprises an objective/contextual rating and a subjective self-report rating of felt response. It also covers two time periods – the day of the event and then two weeks after the start. The *characteristics* of events such as loss and danger are rated regardless of domain for those events with a high level of severity. In addition, there is a scale for the *focus* of the event (on self, jointly with close other, or close other alone), also for the date of the event and for the *independence* of the event (independent of personal action, possibly independent, dependent or disorder-related). This latter occurs when the event can be seen as part of the depression itself, for example, a suicide attempt or being sectioned in a psychiatric hospital. See Figure 1.4.

Difficulties or long-term problems are also assessed in the LEDS (see Figure 1.5). These are problematic circumstances which are continuous for at least four weeks, but most continue for months, some for years. They are rated in the same domains as the life events (e.g. education, health, work) and on a four-point contextual severity scale (where the lowest point still indicates an observable level of difficulty). Such difficulties, particularly at marked level indicate an

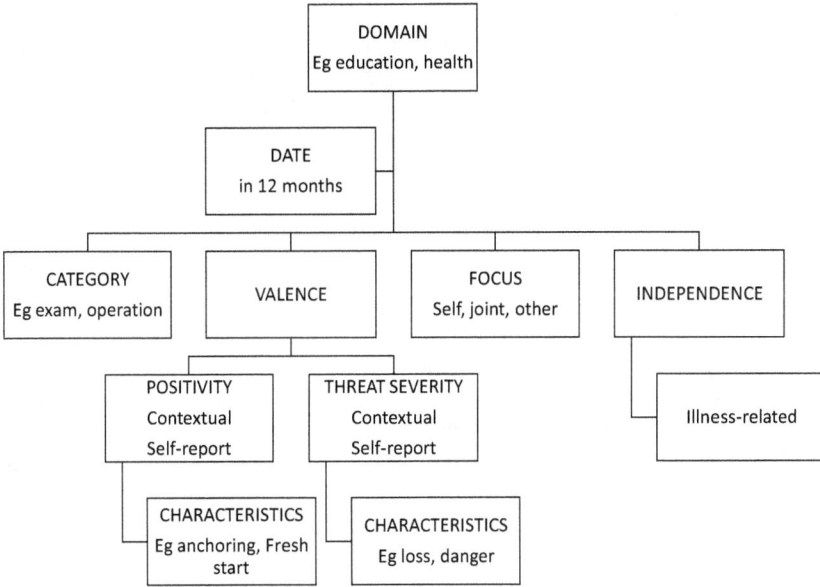

Figure 1.4 Characteristics of life events.

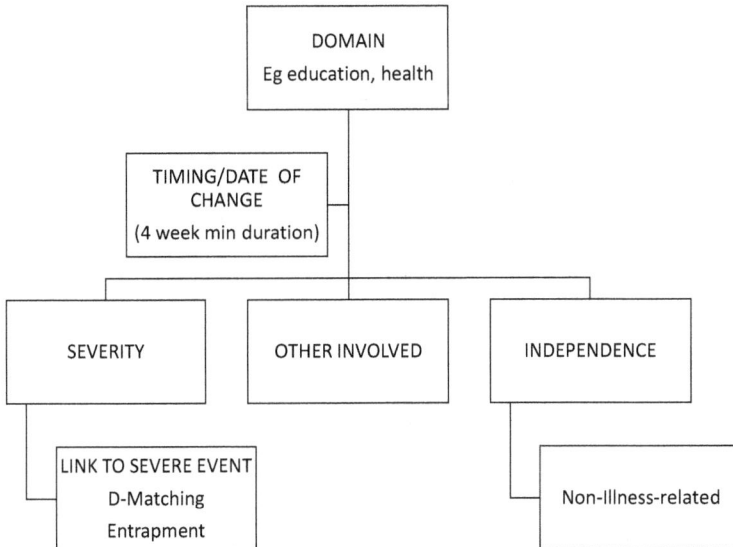

Figure 1.5 Characteristics of difficulties.

accumulation of stress and have the capability of creating life events which sustain the difficulty. For example, a health difficulty around cancer diagnosis will lead to events around diagnosis, hospital operations, radiotherapy or chemotherapy, with potential for remission (and lessening of difficulty) but also worsening of the cancer spread (increasing difficulty). Whilst high-marked difficulties alone are unusual in provoking an episode of depression, they add to the toxicity of severe life events when matched to them (D-matching event). For example, in the health example learning that a treatment has failed and a tumour has returned or grown would constitute a difficulty matching severe life event. This equates with a lessening of hope and an exhaustion of coping strategies. Such D-events increase the likelihood of depression occurring.

The LEDS interview and scoring takes an investigative approach, whereby the *researcher* determines the event ratings based on the account given by the respondent, according to precedent ratings. This is different from measures where the respondent scores their own events as present or stressful. The severity rating (also known as threat/unpleasantness) identifies those which are provoking agents, rated according to pre-established thresholds of events considered distressing to most individuals and rated as high on the scale. Using the LEDS and associated research, we focus in this book on key findings concerning life events that can result in clinical depression.

A key element to be discussed in the book is the issue of how life events are conceptualised and measured and why this is important for both research and clinical practice (see Chapters 5 and 6). Detail, we believe, is necessary in understanding the nature of events and their expected impact on individuals and requires an in-depth approach, such as by interview. The other measurement options available are checklists, which we argue are overly summarised and too proscriptive in outlining the events deemed relevant. These measures we argue are atheoretical and often lead to inconclusive results (see Chapter 5). However, a new online computerised approach, which goes some way to bridge the self-report and investigator-based approaches, is also introduced in Chapter 6.

The next part of this chapter explores the range of life events explored in this book in terms of those extreme, trauma events, comprising threats to life or violence. Given trauma events are highlighted in disorders such as Post-Traumatic Stress Disorder (PTSD) and feature in certain national catastrophic events, these will be highlighted separately (see Chapter 3).

Trauma events

Some severe life events, when extreme, constitute trauma events. Trauma is an ambiguous term, since it covers both the traumatic event or circumstance and the impact of traumatisation on the individual. With regard to the trauma events, these are defined in the Diagnostic and Statistical Manual of Mental Disorders (DSM) as those involving threats to life, violence or sexual violence (APA, 2013). They can also include witness experience including experiences of emergency services personnel who may be called to attend the aftermath of a catastrophic event involving violence or death such as a fire or a terrorist attack. These events are particularly related to PTSD, but also related to emotional disorder such as depression and anxiety (Brewin, 2001). Some trauma events can occur in regular life (e.g. neighbourhood or partner violence; suicide of close other) whilst others are features of natural disasters (e.g. bush fires, floods) including our current worldwide Covid-19 pandemic or accident (e.g. train or airplane crashes). Some occur in the context of war or refugee scenarios. Such events are included in the scope of severe life events and can be differentiated from remaining severe life events and often entail the most marked severity ratings. These are discussed in more detail in Chapter 3.

PTSD is a less common disorder than depression (around 4% affected yearly) but is intrinsically tied to events which constitute a threat to life or violence (Anders, Frazier, & Frankfurt, 2011). This disorder is largely determined by involuntary over-remembering (e.g. nightmares, flashbacks) or under-remembering (amnesia) of the traumatic event, together with negative emotional and cognitive impacts. Its prevalence is 7% over the lifetime (Kessler, Chiu, Demler, Merikangas, & Walters, 2005). It is, however, higher in populations in war conflict zones or among refugees who have suffered more of such experiences (Boscarino & Adams, 2009). It frequently co-exists with depression and has some common origins such as in childhood trauma. This is discussed further in Chapter 3.

Positive experience and wellbeing

Individuals experience as many positive events as negative, and these are shown as potentially aiding recovery from depression or increasing wellbeing states (see Chapters 7 and 8). There are a series of studies from the Bedford Square team showing the impact of positive events prior to recovery/improvement of depression and their characteristics which predict the amelioration of anxiety or depression (Brown, Lemyre, & Bifulco, 1992). The team also examined impacts of positive predisposing features such as positive evaluation of self in this process. This is a finding of potentially high value to psychological interventions and therapies and may benefit from this further dissemination to practitioners. A key element is whether an individual can process and emotionally respond to positive event impacts, particularly if they still retain vulnerability status.

Subjective wellbeing is commonly understood to be the umbrella term which describes how people experience the quality of their life. It includes both cognitive aspects such as positive meaning in life or evaluation of life satisfaction or optimism and emotional aspects such as positive affect of pleasure or joy. It has also been linked to positive relationships and positive beliefs of self, others and the future. Thus, a positive cognitive triad, in Beckian terms (Seligman, 2011). Wellbeing is considered much less episodic than depression and associated more with personality or enduring personal characteristics and robustness. Studies show that positive life events are associated with increases in level of wellbeing (McCullough, Huebner, & Laughlin, 2000). They also lessen the effect of negative life events on depression (Dixon & Reid, 2011) and help in the remission of both depression and anxiety (Brown et al., 1992). In fact, depressed individuals respond to positive events with larger changes in affect, cognition and symptoms than non-depressed individuals and those who have more severe depression have the greatest changes (Khazanov, Ruscio, & Swendsen, 2019). Chapter 8 will outline the relationship of positive events to wellbeing.

Clinical disorder

Whilst the focus of the book is on life events and how they affect mental health, we need to briefly describe the clinical disorders encompassed in the key studies described from the Bedford Square team. We have talked about depression and anxiety as well as PTSD but without explaining that for clinicians this implies not only a type of disorder, but a particular level of severity of symptoms. Throughout this book, we will examine the link between severe life events, vulnerability and emotional disorder, mainly at clinical disorder levels. This encompasses major depression and anxiety states as identified by DSM categories (APA, 2013). As described, the studies mainly use clinical interviews (the Present State Examination – PSE (Wing, Cooper, & Sartorius, 2012) or the Structured Clinical Interview for DSM – SCID (First, Gibbon, Spitzer, & Williams, 1996)).

Just as we argue later that life events are conceptualised with greater validity in detailed measurement, so it is with clinical disorder. The clinical tradition requires a face-to-face interview with a client to establish the array of symptoms which are present, as well as those absent, and their intensity, duration and overlap, to diagnose clinical disorder. Symptom questionnaires were originally designed as a means of screening to identify those for whom an interview would be necessary for diagnosis. But over time, the symptom questionnaires have taken on a life of their own because of ease of administration, providing a total item score to indicate disorder. However, symptom questionnaires do not differentiate well between clinical levels of disorder and subclinical levels, and this can be critical to theoretical models developed. Thus, a number of people may experience minor depression at a less severe level than major depression and with less urgency of treatment. In some circumstances, the former may also indicate a level of resilience if an individual manages to avert a more severe episode. The model of depression developed in this book is specifically about the higher level of clinical disorder such as major depression. Additionally, in modelling the causes of depression, including the role of severe life events, it is critical to get the timing of the onset of disorder to establish the expected sequence. Similarly, for examining recovery (see the Chapter 7 on positive events), it is also critical to establish when symptoms reduce, falling below clinical level or back to normal levels. An outline of major depression symptoms is given below. It should also be noted that the duration of a major depression can be key. Thus, there is literature to show that chronic depression (lasting 12 months or longer) or recurring depression may be a different type of phenomenon from a single acute onset (Brown et al., 2013). Here, the role of vulnerability – or personal susceptibility – may have greater association with such disorder. Thus, there is a potential for anomalous findings when the acute and chronic or recurrent types of depression are not differentiated.

Major depression, as defined in DSM-5,[7] involves the individual experiencing five or more symptoms during the same two-week period where at least one of the symptoms should be either (i) depressed mood or (ii) loss of interest or pleasure. These need to be present 'most of the day, nearly every day'. In addition, other symptoms include significant weight loss or gain, slowing down of thought and reduction of physical movement, fatigue or loss of energy. Also, feelings of worthlessness or guilt, diminished ability to think or concentrate, or indecisiveness, or recurrent thoughts of death, suicidal ideation a suicide attempt are also symptoms considered in major depression diagnosis. These symptoms must cause the individual clinically significant distress or impairment in social, occupational or other important areas of functioning to be counted as reaching clinical levels of disorder.

Anxiety is rather more complicated because it has different forms.[8] Maybe the best known is panic and/or agoraphobia, two disorders which frequently co-exist – the first indicating overwhelming fear including autonomic symptoms which come on unexpectedly or are triggered by certain situations, and the latter the avoidance of situations, particularly travelling and open spaces. Other disorders are Generalised Anxiety Disorder characterised by overwhelming worry, even about small things, and Social Phobia/Social Anxiety disorder which is a fear of social situations including eating or speaking in public and performing.[9] These are the disorders subsumed under clinical anxiety as described in Chapters 2 and 7. (Neither common phobia nor obsessional compulsive disorder is included in the studies described there.) Anxiety frequently co-exists with depression (50% with depression also have anxiety), often indicating a more chronic trajectory, and it is also related to severe life events. As with depression, anxiety is treatable with medication and/or therapy (Carleton, Peluso, Collimore, & Asmundson, 2011).

Major depression is a debilitating disorder which can have impacts on an individual's work (through loss of concentration or time off sick), relationships (through irritability or social withdrawal) or parenting (through loss of interest and tiredness). It affects around 10% of people per year (Hasin et al., 2018) with a lifetime prevalence of 20–28% (Vandeleur et al., 2017). It is twice as common in women as men and occurs more in working-class groups and those socially excluded.[10] It is a common disorder internationally and now ranked by WHO as one of the major health problems worldwide estimated to affect 350 million people and is the leading cause of disability worldwide in terms of total years lost due to disability.[11] Prevalence is increasing with depression rates rising globally by one-fifth from 2005 to 2015, and researchers found that people born after 1945 were ten times likely to struggle with a depressive disorder than people born before 1945 (Smith & Rutter, 1995).[12] Another unintuitive phenomenon is that the wealthier a country the higher the rates of depression. Depression is however treatable, with both medication and psychotherapy being effective. The psychological treatments most advocated in the UK are Cognitive Behavioural Therapies (CBT) which are relatively brief and focused on changing both cognitions and behaviours with a focus on current circumstances and vulnerabilities, but other psychotherapies are also effective (see Chapter 8 for more details). Medication is also a common treatment pathway.

The studies by the Bedford Square team referred to in this book mainly use London community-based samples, many of them involving women (see Appendix 1 for an outline of the studies whose results are discussed in this book). The rationale for this is that emotional disorder such as depression has a high prevalence rate in the community – for example, around 10% (using clinical interview approaches) and the risk of relapse is high with 50% relapsing after the first episode and 70%, after the second episode with rates double in women (Girgus & Yang, 2015). Thus, it is a commonly experienced disorder and can be captured in community samples as well as in psychiatric patients.

Reasons for the higher rates of depression in women have been explored. Whist various biological interpretations have been considered, gender roles and the different types of life events and gender-based coping styles are argued to play a significant part. A study of over a thousand community-based adults found that women were more likely to experience chronic negative circumstances, to have a lower sense of mastery and to engage more in ruminative coping than men (Nolen-Hoeksema, Larson, & Grayson, 1999). A further study of the types of events which affected women more than men was studied in 100 London cohabiting couples screened for the presence of a shared severe life event and focused on looking at gender differences in response (Nazroo, Edwards, & Brown, 1997). It found that women had a greater risk of a depressive episode following the shared life event than men with the greater risk entirely restricted to events involving children, housing or reproductive problems which had greater day-to-day impact on the women. In addition, it was found that this occurred more among couples where there were clear traditional gender differences in associated roles. This was explained by women reporting feeling more responsible for these domestic events whilst men distanced themselves more. Once child crises were excluded in the analysis, the rates of depression between the genders were similar. The hypothesis that men respond with more anger which buffers against depression was not upheld – women too expressed anger at events (Nazroo, Edwards, & Brown, 1998).

Whilst we will not demonstrate a major cultural focus in this book, culture is relevant both to frequency and type of life events, to the support available and to rates of emotional disorder. The work of James Nazroo and colleagues has examined disorder in Black, Asian and Minority Ethnic groups and shown high rates alongside discriminatory experience (Karlsen, Nazroo, McKenzie, Bhui, & Weich, 2005; Sproston & Nazroo, 2002). A complementary approach has looked at the life events and depression models across varied cultures internationally and found replications, for example, in Africa (Broadhead & Abas, 1998) and Pakistan (Chaudhry, Husain, Tomenson, & Creed, 2012).

Clinical implications of life events

Most professionals in the clinical field today would accept that severe life events are causally related to disorders such as depression, anxiety and PTSD. This is not only because models such as CBT build identifying the provoking events into the therapy process, but because clients in distress will usually describe the circumstances that have caused them such pain. But many clinicians will be less aware of subtleties of how life events can be categorised and assessed, the extent to which they impinge on human need due to specific characteristics and the extent to which they can reflect common environmental pressures. This is in part because medical models which highlight biological vulnerability have strong influence in psychiatric treatment and in part because of cognitive models which highlight the individual's susceptibility and influence psychological therapies. Both tend to underestimate the social context which can explain emotional disorder in communities or groups.

However, another reason is because the knowledge and importance of event dimensions may not have sufficiently percolated through to therapeutic practice. This may be because of short cuts taken in recent research measurement diverging from intensive interview approaches to rely on checklist questionnaires. This has tended to treat life events as a standard listing, devoid of context, personal circumstance and timing, and amenable to an analysis only by means of an overall cumulative score. In such measurement schemes, this means that a rape could be given a single scoring equivalent to a move of house and thus underestimated in terms of its toxicity. We argue that checklists are over-condensed and underestimate the true number and severity of events for the individual (see Chapter 5). The message has thus been perpetuated that life events are somehow regular life changes (house move is often cited as the worse type of life change) and that the number of events rather than the nature of events has most impact on disorder. For practitioners, this therefore loses the theoretical linkages to psychological need, vulnerability and the social context. In fact, it only takes one toxic severe life event to provoke a clinical depression. Understanding which event is the most likely to provoke a depression or anxiety state could be of great help to clinician formulations.

Clinicians are of course aware of the role of stressful events in triggering disorder. Therapies such as CBT or counselling often begin with questioning about the recent changes in life circumstances to look for crises that might have triggered a strong emotional reaction leading to disorder. Usually, a therapist will focus on the situation presented by the client – maybe a death, divorce or finance problem. Thus, they are reliant on a subjective account which may be influenced by individual vulnerability or some tunnel vision affected by their symptoms. Yet from what we have seen in interview-based measures compared to checklists, the extent of the crisis – or stressful event – can be under-reported. If all the negative circumstances were identified, together with full context and clustering of events and longer-term problems, the clinician might reassess the individual's actual vulnerability or in fact resilience in relation to the distress experienced. Those who study events know that there is a frequent clustering of both related events (e.g. marital discord, marital separation and housing crisis) and unrelated events – for example, an elderly parent's death coinciding with an employment difficulty, bullying at work or child's delinquency. Coping with one such problem may well be within an individual's capabilities, but trying to cope with several at once can tax even those with robust coping skills. We hope our explication of the complexity of events and their measurement will aid clinical psychologists and psychotherapists in making their assessments to get as full a picture as possible of life circumstances and the likely precipitating factors for emotional disorder. Throughout this book, the implications for clinical practice are drawn out and interventions which we consider linked to the theoretical model developed (see Chapters 7 and 8).

We hope that this elucidation of life events as the way in which people can be affected by their experience will lead to a greater understanding of psychological disorder which puts weight on people's misfortunes rather than their 'weakness'. In this way, we hope to counter some of the stigma attached to clinical disorder and have people understand how individuals succumb to life events with particular juxtaposition of circumstance and individual history and psychology. In this way, we hope to contribute to current policies which seek to improve quality of life of people in the UK and internationally through better understanding and better focusing of intervention.

Notes

1 https://www.britannica.com/biography/John-Graunt
2 https://booth.lse.ac.uk/map
3 https://www.britannica.com/event/Chernobyl-disaster
4 https://www.imdb.com/title/tt7366338
5 https://www.bbc.com/news/world-australia-50951043
6 https://www.fwi.co.uk/news/suicide-stats-exceed-bse-deaths
7 https://www.psycom.net/depression-definition-dsm-5-diagnostic-criteria/
8 https://www.psychiatry.org/patients-families/anxiety-disorders/what-are-anxiety-disorders
9 https://www.halffullnotempty.com/dsm-5-anxiety-disorders/
10 https://www.nice.org.uk/guidance/TA367/documents/major-depressive-disorder-vortioxetine-id583-final-scope2
11 https://www.who.int/mental_health/management/depression/wfmh_paper_de-pression_wmhd_2012.pdf
12 https://pulsetms.com/resources/around-world

Section 1

Life events and depression

2 Life events are multi-dimensional

There is a substantial link between severe life events and psychological disorder. However, the research on the characteristics of specific life events to identify first what makes them severe and second what makes them highly impactful for particular individuals is less well known. This is approached in two ways in this chapter: first, identifying how severe events can threaten human needs and provide potential for psychological and emotional damage, and second, identifying characteristics of severe events which challenge or threaten particular needs. This moves towards a multi-dimensional understanding of how life events impact on an individual's life.

The term 'life event' has become a catchall for a variety of life experiences not always well-defined. This can encompass daily hassles, normative life change, disruptive change and that related to longer-term chronic problems and significant change that can be either positive or negative. Part of the confusion has been due to the operational definitions of a life event. We consider the following to encapsulate the nature of a live event:

> An acute change to roles, relationships, routines or material or health circumstances as part of the social or physical environment. It can provide a challenge to coping and adaptation. It encompasses both normative and non-normative change and its valence can extend from positive or mildly negative to very negative, encompassing trauma experience. It can be focused on the individual/self or to those close. It has both an objective aspect around what has happened, as well as a subjective aspect of how the individual interprets its meaning.

Definitions utilised in the Life Events and Difficulties Schedule (LEDS) emphasise a number of important elements of life events that are considered severe and act on the aetiology of disorder as seen in the quote below:

> The research literature on general life stress and depression suggests that the most etiologically relevant stressful life events are (a) acute (i.e. distinct onset), (b) very recent (within approximately 3 to 6 months), (c) major (i.e. very threatening or unpleasant), and (d) primarily focused on the participant (i.e. the event directly affects the participant; Brown & Harris, 1978).
>
> (Monroe & Reid, 2008, p. 951)

Life events are extraordinarily varied, in terms of category, and in the LEDS interview, there are ten or more, each with an additional ten or so subcategories, thus over 100 varieties of event. However, there are other elements besides category. Some life events appear to be about more normative changes – such as leaving school, getting a job, moving in with a partner or retiring. These events are usually relevant to life stages and have a planned or predictable element to them. However, events that seem normative can still be negative in some circumstances when the individual has less control (e.g. forced retirement without adequate pension funds). Other life events seem more inherently challenging to negative life change, such as untimely death of someone close, illness or severe financial loss. The extent to which a life event is negative cannot necessarily be prejudged by its label and can be dependent upon individual circumstances or context. Assessing negativity is important for understanding how the event links to psychological disorder. Some negative events such as bereavement or diagnosis of cancer can be assumed to be highly threatening for most people. But other events – such as redundancy, pregnancy, divorce – may vary in their negativity or positivity according to circumstances. People also experience positive life events which bring about positive change, such as creating a new role, realising a worked-for goal or reducing a prior negative situation involving difficulty or deprivation. These also depend upon context. For example, a pregnancy event may be highly positive for someone who has been trying to get pregnant for years, but highly negative for someone when it is the result of rape. Just as negative life events have implications for psychological disorder, positive life events have implications for increased wellbeing.

Sequences of events

Life events are acute and therefore can be dated to the day they occur. For example, being diagnosed with a serious health condition is a discrete life event which can be dated to the first time the individual is given the diagnosis. However, if that event continues to impact the person for several months, then it is likely to bring up additional life events (e.g. hospital stays, operations) all of which may be severe i.e. significant and negative. The underlying health problem then is termed an ongoing difficulty (or long-term problem) in LEDS. Similarly, an individual may have an ongoing minor difficulty with a live-in partner characterised by tension and infrequent arguments. A severe event of more significance may then occur such as a major argument (including threat of separation or violence) or an actual separation with one member leaving the household. This may then heighten the severity of the underlying relationship problem, for example, involving child custody or finances. Events are thus at times linked to such underlying difficulties. This allows for developing interesting indices in the LEDS combining measurement scales (of severe event and ongoing difficulty) which can add to prediction of disorder.

Most studies of life events and their capacity to provoke emotional disorder use a 12-month time period of study. This is long enough to capture an episode of disorder in the time frame and also allows for documentation of some weeks prior to onset for the events to be examined. It is also a recent enough period for the individual to recall most of what has happened in detail. Such research has found a relatively small time gap between a severe life event and onset of depression of under 12 weeks (Brown, Bifulco, & Andrews, 1990a). Ascertaining some precision of dating of events and difficulties is therefore necessary in testing a causal relationship.

The life events and difficulties schedule (LEDS)

Research in the 1970s–1990s provided for a rich tradition in the UK of investigating life events intensively by interview to explain social class differences in emotional disorder (e.g. Brown & Harris, 1978; Goodyer, 1995; Paykel, 1997). This favoured the use of complex semi-structured interviews and narrative approaches, whereby features of an event coupled with the individuals' particular life context could be assessed. This intensive approach proved to be more predictive of disorder than questionnaire approaches and better at capturing life events in general (Donoghue, Traviss-Turner, House, Lewis, & Gilbody, 2016; McQuaid et al., 1992) and their response to environmental adversity (Harkness & Monroe, 2016) (see Chapter 5 for more details). The LEDS, a semi-structured interview, has long been considered the 'gold standard' in life events measurement (op cit).

The theoretical basis of LEDS differs from checklists in several fundamental ways. The original checklists were based on the assumption that it is the *accumulation* of life stress which puts an individual at risk for physical or mental ill health. In other words, a total score of the number of life events in a period of time is created and the higher the score the higher the depression rate. In contrast, for an onset of major depression, the LEDS utilises a method where individual severe events are examined in relation to onset of disorder, with one event in particular is identified, as particularly impactful for that individual and context and usually closest to onset. Other models have examined events of lesser severity as potentially provoking, this particularly in psychiatric patients who have become highly sensitised due to recurrent episodes, known as the kindling hypothesis (Post, 1992). The LEDS approach assesses all events, and some studies have shown that even non severe events can be predictive of disorders such as bipolar disorder (Kemner, Mesman, Nolen, Eijckemans, & Hillegers, 2015) showing the utility of scoring all events including those less negative.

The LEDS comprises categories of ten life domains including education, housing, money, crime, health, fertility and reproduction, marital, other relationships, death and miscellaneous. It's time coverage is usually the 12-month period prior to interview, sometimes extended slightly earlier to allow for the match between a severe event and six-month difficulty at the beginning of the period. (This is described later in this chapter.) Within each domain are numerous subcategories of events, questioned about during the interview. When an event (or life change) is identified, interviewers question about the facts of the event in detail to establish sufficient context to rate the severity of the event for that person. This is repeated in each domain until a comprehensive picture of the year has been attained. The interview covers events to the self as well as to a predetermined list of close family and confidants. The interview is audio-recorded to enable the interview flow without pauses for writing down information, and ratings are made later (in the office) for each event and difficulty identified. These are located within a calendar to check for dates and sequences. Ratings of threat or severity of events are determined on a precedent rating, with manualised examples, with those in doubt discussed at consensus meetings where researchers meet to discuss complex ratings. Interviews take around an hour, but rating and finalising take two and half times as long. Due to the comprehensive and precise nature of the LEDS, anyone wishing to use it must attend a training course.[1]

A key rating for determining severity of a life events using the LEDS method is that of 'threat/unpleasantness' (see Figure 2.1 for scales rated). This includes negative characteristics of the event which challenge basic needs, as ascertained for the average individual in that situation or context. Threat is rated for two time periods – when it first happened/the following day (*short-term threat*) and after 10–14 days later (*long-term threat*. A rating is made of *contextual threat* which is an objective or factual rating which considers the relevant background information to the life event *in situ* and its anticipated consequences, judging how severe that would be for the average person). A rating is then made for the *reported threat* using the same scaling which reflects the individual's emotional account and reported reactions to the life event. For many, the rating of reported and contextual will be the same, unless there is evidence of 'over-reporting' (catastrophising or

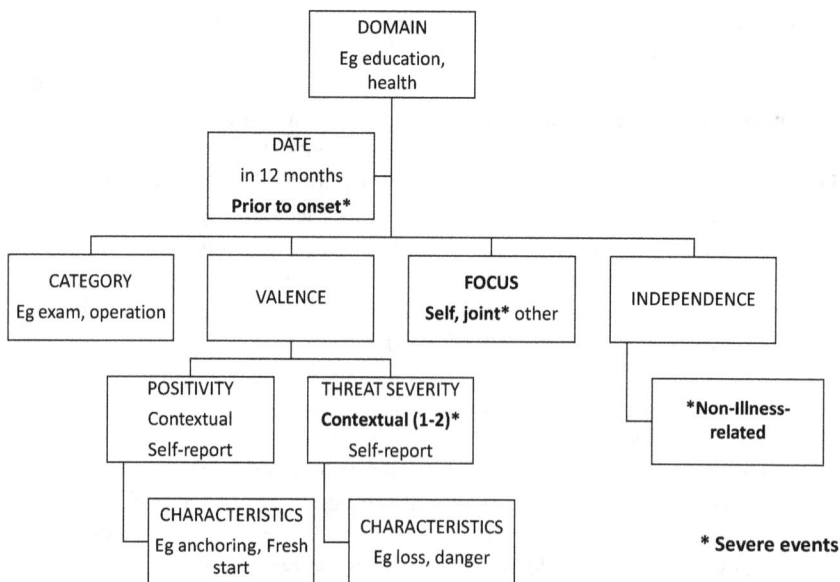

Figure 2.1 Characteristics of life events – highlighting severe events.

emotionally volatile account) or 'under-reporting' (downplaying or denial of the event significance). *Contextual factors* and how these impact on the event scoring can include any that increase the threat unpleasantness of the event, for example, for pregnancy, it could include financial concerns, ongoing relationship difficulties, housing problems, cultural and religious norms or stigma and community values, which explicate the meaning of the event for that individual.

Severe life event

Severe event is the name for an event which can provoke an episode of depression. Critical to this classification are the following: first, the *contextual threat* level must be scored as 'marked' or 'moderate' (1–2) on a 4-point scale and is based on the long-term (two-weekly) as opposed to the short-term (immediate) threat level. The second precondition is the focus of the event (to whom the event happens), given that events to those close family and confidants are also included in the LEDS questioning. In the rating system, events can be categorised as those which happen mainly to the participant (*self-focused*), together with someone close (*joint-focused*) or only to the close other (*other-focused*). If the event was either *self-focused* or *joint-focused*, then the event meets criteria for a severe event. The only exception to this rule is for those extremely negative events (rated as a '1 marked' and often involving trauma or bereavement) which are automatically rated as severe regardless of the focus. A third factor which affects the rating is whether the event is independent of the outcome variable of study (i.e. psychological disorder-related). This is included to avoid circularity in research studies. For example, if an individual had an event such as suicide attempt, and depression was the study outcome, the event would be rated but excluded from analysis as a potential provoking agent. This is to avoid aspects of the depression itself being counted as an external event which can provoke the disorder.

Examples of severe life events

Examples of severe life events selected from research interviews are included below. Details of the individual's perceptions or reported threat of the event are also included:

* Death of mother from cancer: this young woman's mother had a breast cancer diagnosis in the mother's late 40s – there is a family history of it, with her grandmother having died young of the same disease. Her mother underwent a year of treatment for which her daughter provided care and support. They had a close relationship. The severe event involved the mother's death. For reported threat – the woman described herself as 'devastated', highly distressed and felt a huge loss in her life. The contextual rating also reflected this ('marked').
* Separation from partner of 12 years: this woman was involved in a partner relationship that had been difficult with months of conflict. The couple

have young children. She was afraid of her partner who bullied her and undermined her self-confidence. He made it difficult for her to have friends and would mock her in front of the children. They had several rows which were heated and hostile. Eventually, she was persuaded to leave him, and the severe life event is when she told him it was over, left the flat and went to live with her mother. Her reported threat was that she was frightened that her husband might find her and worried about the future for herself and her children. This was also reflected on the contextual rating ('marked'). On the positive side, she also felt a strong sense of relief and was proud of the move she had made.

- Evicted from home: this single mother was evicted from her social housing due to inability to pay the rent. She is forced to take her young children to live in bed and breakfast accommodation with no cooking facilities or play area. The lack of rent payment was due to underlying financial difficulties given she was reliant on benefits and unable to work whilst her youngest child was still a baby and her older child in nursery for only short hours. She contacted social services who arranged the accommodation. It is in a deprived area and has insufficient facilities. When she reported the threat experienced, she describes it as awful leaving the flat; she felt she had failed her children and is pessimistic about how she is going to find a comfortable and safe place for them to live whilst living on benefits. The reported threat was rated at the same level as the contextual threat ('moderate'). Although this was clearly a highly disruptive event, it did not have the level of danger from violence or finality of loss of the two events described earlier.

- Adolescent child attacked by a neighbourhood gang: this mother had been unaware of her teenage son being bullied. He had come home with injuries he claimed were accidental but had showed signs of anxiety and withdrawal. The event involves an attack by a gang of aggressive youth where he is both very frightened and has injuries. When she reported the threat of this event, she described that she had not been aware that her son was under stress and had not really noticed his changed behaviour. She minimised and felt little distress. She reported that bullying happens in adolescence and generally people get over it. Therefore, the reported threat ('some') was rated lower than contextual threat ('moderate').

- Loss of job with serious financial implications: this man is the family wage earner, and he lost his job during the financial recession after the banking crash in 2007. There was no specific warning. There is little prospect of finding another suitable job in his field as an estate agent given the slump in the housing market. The couple have three children to support as well as a mortgage to pay. When reporting the threat of the event, he explained that he had been reluctant to tell his wife about it because he didn't want to worry her. In fact, he didn't tell her about the event for two weeks after it happened because he thought he might be able to find something else and didn't think it was too problematic. He still thinks he will find something and has delayed any new financial planning since he doesn't want other people to know about it. He thinks that it will all work out fine. Thus, his reported rating of threat ('some') was lower than the contextual rating ('moderate').

Difficulties are rated similarly in LEDS, but on fewer scales (see Figure 2.2). In the above examples, all but the last one followed ongoing problem situations which existed prior to the event. Thus, ratings include the ten overall categories utilised for events (e.g. health, education, partner), the persons involved in the difficulty, and then objective severity is scored on a 4-point scale – where the lowest point still indicates some level of problem. The severity rating is open to change over time, and the initial point of the difficulty and the change points are all recorded by date. A simplified system rates the peak of the difficulty rather than all the change points. Marked difficulties are those rated 1–3 (marked, high-moderate or low-moderate) on the severity scale and are non-health related. Difficulties rarely contribute alone as provoking agents for disorder, but their main role is in contributing to the generation of severe life events, but also in creating an added dimension to severe life events where they precede and 'match' the difficulty domain of the event thereby increasing risk of depression. In the examples above all but the last involve D-matching events where an event matches an existing difficulty. Thus, the severe life event is effectively in a sequence following the longer-term difficulty which makes it likely to lead to an exhaustion of coping or diminution of hope in the individual. It can also lead to situations of entrapment (see later in this chapter).

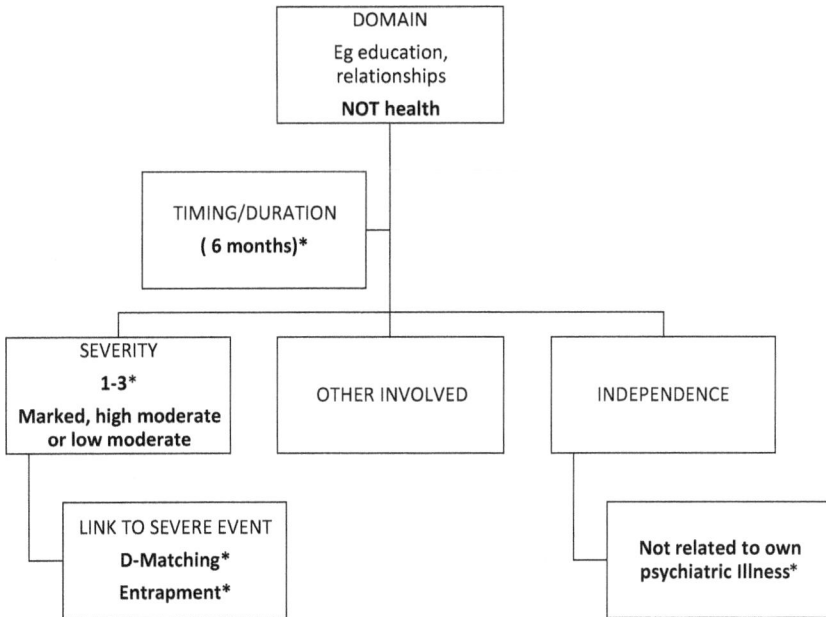

Figure 2.2 Characteristics of difficulties – highlighting matching.

Updating life events and reflecting cultural issues

The LEDS is a highly comprehensive measure and works on a case-by-case basis to provide detailed ratings of events and difficulties according to the principles expounded above. The categories occasionally need updating to keep pace with modern life, culture and technology. Thus, technological events (such as trolling, identity stealing, cyberbullying and online grooming) have been included in the more recent online version of the measure (CLEAR – see Chapter 6). Due to increasing world globalisation and connectivity through media and travel, events which take place on one side of the world can impact on those on the other side of the world, and these are taken into account in 'geopolitical events'. Even within the realm of health and fertility, unforeseen advances mean new types of life events (e.g. through IVF) now exist that were not included in the original measure. As life expectancy increases and the medical field progresses so to do the number and range of health life events. Although people live longer due to these advances, they and their families may deal with more chronic disease which can include novel treatments of an invasive nature. Similarly, with increased air travel, epidemics can become pandemics and affect more people worldwide. As this book is being written, the pandemic of coronavirus means that people all over the world have been affected by it creating a plethora of personal life events new in this particular context. A tool such as the LEDS is sufficiently flexible to allow for such updates and amendments.

Events involving cultural issues are also capable of being included in the LEDS scoring system by adjusting for cultural context. For example, the context to a marriage may include one arranged by parents, forced on an unwilling young person or even in some cultures being taken as the second wife. This context would be included in the threat rating. Another culturally specific context maybe a woman considering a termination due to financial and marital difficulties but be unable to ask for support because of her religious affiliation and the stigma involved within her community. This again is taken into account and can raise the threat rating. When assessing circumstances such as marital separation in Moslem countries, this can include stigma and rejection of the woman by the community, even when the husband caused the separation (Abdul Kadir & Bifulco, 2011). It can also include another wife joining the family without the first wife's consent. These important details can be included in the threat rating and the difficulty resulting.

Additional event dimensions

In order to guide the decision-making around the critical threat/unpleasantness rating, other relevant event aspects can be invoked as a rating guide to inform understanding. This encapsulates the generic underlying dimensions related to human need which can cut across domain categories (such as education or finance) and challenge psychological wellbeing and require psychological adaptation. The different characteristics of life events captured in the LEDS such as loss and danger or D-matching events are now described in more detail throughout the rest of this chapter. The relative importance of the event itself and its appraisal reflects the differentiation between the socio-environmental influence (involving, e.g. poverty or deprivation) versus individual cognitive characteristics (involving, e.g. low self-esteem or pessimism). This further develops the personalised response to events which link prior cognitive vulnerability. In the next section, we focus on these different characteristics along with a summary of the research by the Bedford Square team and how it may provide a key to understanding the 'severe' in life events.

Loss and danger events

There is a long tradition associating loss with depression. Thus, equating the experience of loss with an event involving death is a natural one. But there are other forms of loss which may be less permanent but also distressing. Separations from close others are also losses, and some can be permanent. Loss, however, spans many different areas, and loss can occur in most domains. For example, job loss, financial loss, loss of physical possessions or home, loss of health, loss of bodily function and so on. Loss has also been encompassed in the cognitive research literature but also extended to evolutionary and adaptive aspects (Beck & Bredemeier, 2016). This more holistic examination of loss is summarised:

> We propose that depression can be viewed as an adaptation to conserve energy after the perceived loss of an investment in a vital resource such as a relationship, group identity, or personal asset. Tendencies to process information negatively and experience strong biological reactions to stress (resulting from genes, trauma, or both) can lead to depressogenic beliefs about the self, world, and future. These tendencies are mediated by alterations in brain areas/networks involved in cognition and emotion regulation. Depressogenic beliefs predispose individuals to make cognitive appraisals that amplify perceptions of loss, typically in response to stressors that impact available resources. (Beck & Bredemeier, 2016) (Abstract)

Brown and Harris noted that many severe events had an element of loss involved. In one of the first papers looking at loss in relation to severe life events, loss was defined as including loss through death or separation of someone close but also loss given a wider remit related to health, possessions, employment or career prospects or a cherished idea (Finlay-Jones & Brown, 1981). This suggests that although loss does happen perhaps more often in the area of 'attachment', such as the death of someone close or loss of a relationship, it can simultaneously affect other basic needs. If someone loses a partner, this may also have an impact on their perceptions of 'security' as they lose a main source of income and on their 'identity' as they have viewed themselves as part of a couple for a number of years. Interestingly, in a note for the criteria for major depression in the DSM 5 (APA, 2013), life events related to some sort of loss (death, financial ruin, medical

illness, disability and losses related to a natural disaster) are acknowledged as being causative for depression. This is not without controversy given bereavement
event-related depression was excluded from the diagnostic criteria in DSM-IV
(Parker, Paterson, & Hadzi-Pavlovic, 2015).

Danger is defined in LEDS as the threat of future loss and is associated with
fear and vigilance. Finlay-Jones and Brown developed a 4-point scale of danger,
grading severe events as having severe danger ('marked' or 'moderate' levels) or
not, similar to how they rated loss (Finlay-Jones & Brown, 1981). Danger in a
severe event was defined as:

> the likelihood of it bringing about future unpleasant crises of a specific future
> crisis which might occur as a result of the event ..... While the future crisis
> stemming from the severe event had to have some probability of occurring
> for the rating of danger, this crisis should not be inevitable. (p. 806), (Finlay-
> Jones & Brown, 1981)

Thus, danger exists where a future crisis is a possibility, but not inevitable.
So, for example, if someone heard by email of father's diagnosis of cancer and
impending death, then this is likely to already be rated as loss because of the
inevitability and short-term expectation. However, if the father had been diagnosed with a serious illness where death was a possibility, but not an immediate
eventuality, then danger would be rated. 'Danger' in a severe event can also go
across domains. Take, for example, the diagnosis of a potential life-threatening
disease in a partner which would have implications for both health and partner
relationship.

Finlay-Jones & Brown looked at severe events involving loss and danger in a London community sample (Finlay-Jones & Brown, 1981) (see study 2, Appendix 1).
A significant association was found between loss in relation to severe life events
and the onset of depression and in relation to mixed anxiety and depression (see
Figure 2.3). Their results show the specificity of type of event in the relationship to
disorder. For individuals with severe loss events, 65% had depression compared to
47% with mixed disorder and only 8% with anxiety (p < 0.001, see Figure 2.3 left-
hand columns). For anxiety disorder, the reverse held. The rates were 62% for danger events, 47% for mixed events and 24% for loss events, respectively (p < 0.001,
Figure 2.3 right-hand columns). For those with mixed depression/anxiety disorder,
33% had mixed disorder compared to 33% depressed and none with anxiety alone
(middle columns Figure 2.3) (Finlay-Jones & Brown, 1981). Therefore, danger was
a predictor of anxiety and loss of depression. Mixed anxiety and depression were
present when events had elements of both loss and danger.

These findings have been replicated in adolescents using an events checklist
approach (Asselmann, Wittchen, Lieb, Hofler, & Beesdo-Baum, 2015). Here,
loss events predicted episodes of 'pure' depression [odds ratio[2] (OR) 2.4, p <
0.001], whereas danger events predicted episodes of 'pure' anxiety (OR 2.3,
p = 0.023) as well as 'pure' depression (OR 2.5, p < 0.001). Mixed events also
predicted both disorders (OR 2.9 and 2.4, respectively) but more importantly

% with clinical disorder

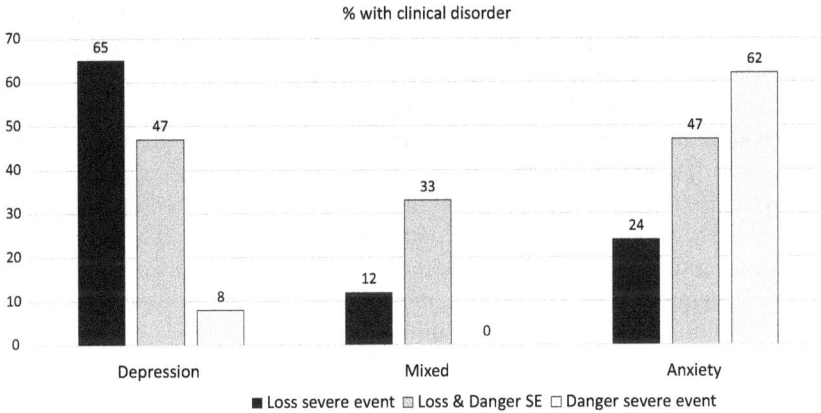

Figure 2.3 Loss and danger events and disorder.

their co-morbidity (OR 3.6, p < 0.001). These dimensions have also been examined in relation to bi-polar depression with loss relating to the depressive phases (Hosang, Uher, Maugham, McGuffin, & Farmer, 2012). The importance of these studies highlighted that dimensions of loss were likely to be more important than the details of the event itself for predicting depression. Although the work looking at loss has shown that it widens the field from just interpersonal loss to other areas, there is a lot of evidence that interpersonal loss is of particular relevance when predicting onset of depression. This has been found in a prospective study of adolescents (Monroe, Rohde, Seeley, & Lewinsohn, 1999) in pregnancy (Asselmann et al., 2015) and in a study focusing on gender differences (Kendler, Gatz, Gardner, & Pedersen, 2006). Interpersonal loss seems to be particularly depressogenic when it involves bereavement (Broadhead & Abas, 1998) and separation when initiated by the close other (Kendler, Hettema, Butera, Gardner, & Prescott, 2003).

Humiliation and entrapment events

Humiliation occurs when a person of higher social status criticises or insults an individual of lower social status (Hartling & Luchetta, 1999). The associated emotion is that of shame. Humiliation has also been defined as 'feeling devalued in relation to others or to a core sense of self, usually with an element of rejection or a sense of role failure' (p. 791) (Kendler et al., 2003). Early study of such loss of status derived from the ethology literature based on social ranking theory in animals (Gilbert, 2000; Price, Sloman, Gardner, Gilbert, & Rohde, 1994). Thus, animals suffer from exclusion or loss of status in the 'pecking order' when challenged by stronger competitors and show signs of submission. A similar process is argued for humans with a likely depressogenic reaction when a person's status, rank or attractiveness is undermined.

Brown and colleagues identified three core areas in their rating of humiliation in relationships – a rejecting separation from a close person; an act of 'delinquency' by someone close, for example, a family member being given a prison sentence considered shaming, or a 'put down' when an individual is embarrassed in public (see Figure 2.4) (Brown, Harris, & Hepworth, 1995). This study, combining community women (Appendix 1, study 3) and depressed patients (study 4) found that loss events which could be further specified as humiliation were three times more likely to lead to depression compared to other types of loss alone (e.g. death or initiated separation) (see Figure 2.5). They concluded that their original definition of loss was too over-arching – the difference between someone leaving a relationship and someone being left by someone else can be critical to humiliation categorisation although both involve loss.

The findings have been further borne out by studies where other-initiated separations are similarly differentiated as humiliations (Farmer & McGuffin, 2003;

Humiliation

'Put-down'

- a woman being told by her husband that she is abnormal (because of her epilepsy) and not fit to be a mother, in a row that led to a marital separation.
- a single mother criticized by a magistrate for failing to keep up payments for a fine incurred by her teenage son and told she could in future be sent to prison.

Separation with failure or rejection

- a 9-year-old daughter who told her mother she wanted to leave her mother and go back to live in the West Indies.
- a 14-year-old daughter who insists to her mother that she will go and live with her estranged father.

Others delinquency

- an adolescent daughter found stealing from her mother's purse and playing truant.

Figure 2.4 Examples of humiliation severe events.

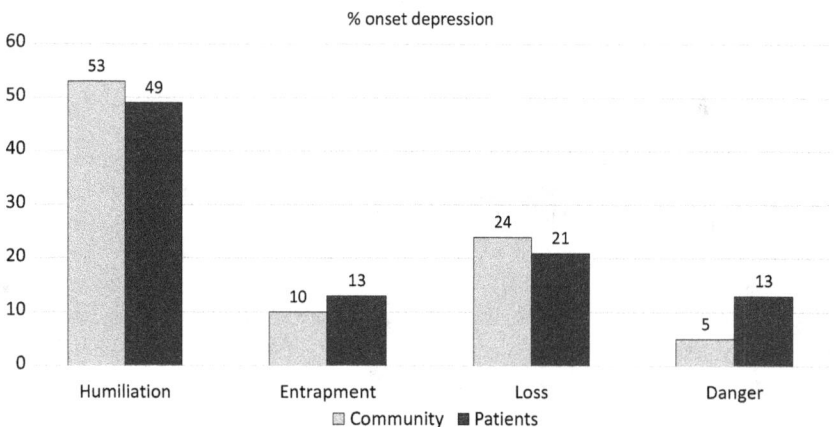

Figure 2.5 Humiliation and entrapment events and depression.

Kendler et al., 2003). Kendler and colleagues, researching in the USA, looked at a large sample of both males and females and rated their events including humiliation scoring for all severe events and not only those that already had severe loss or danger (Kendler et al., 2003). They found that loss and humiliation predicted depression independently of one another suggesting that each dimension inflicts a different aspect of emotional damage. Humiliation as an element of severe events did not predict anxiety alone but did predict an onset of comorbid anxiety and depression. Danger showed a similar relationship to mixed disorder. In addition, they found that other-initiated separations as a subset of humiliation were particularly likely to be related to depression. Similar findings were reported by Parker and colleagues (Parker et al., 2015). Another type of event which was rated consistently as involving humiliation is having a family member who has committed a criminal offence (Collazzoni et al., 2015) which also fits with definitions above (Siddaway, Taylor, Wood, & Schulz, 2015).

Investigating the role of humiliation in individuals at the unipolar depressed phase of a bipolar disorder, humiliation (along with loss and danger) was found to be significantly related to depression. However, the investigators noted that danger is also related to depression, but the study did not measure anxiety to look for potential comorbidity (Hosang et al., 2012). The finding that humiliation is an important feature of severe events has not been limited to westernised societies but was also studied in a sample of women in Zimbabwe with similar results (Broadhead & Abas, 1998).

Humiliation is also associated with entrapment and defeat. Defeat has been looked at in the animal literature based on the social ranking theories referred to above. When an animal is being threatened and is likely to lose the encounter, it engages in short-term strategies in order to protect itself. This has been called Involuntary Defeat Syndrome (IDS) which allows the animal to protect itself from further harm (Price et al., 1994). The animal becomes socially withdrawn, sleeps less, eats less and increases its hypervigilance. When the threat is no longer there, the IDS deactivates and the animal returns to its normal state. If there is no available escape for the animal, it will engage in a further defensive strategy called 'arrested flight' (Dixon, Fisch, Huber, & Walser, 1989) where it disengages from its environment by a display of submissive behaviours (Griffiths, Wood, Maltby, Taylor, & Tai, 2014). These patterns of IDS and 'arrested flight' have been linked to patterns of human psychopathology. Defeat in humans is a failed struggle which is not just limited to the social sphere as with animals (Sturman & Mongrain, 2006) and is viewed as different to loss (Taylor, Gooding, Wood, & Tarrier, 2011). Related to this is entrapment or the inability to escape a highly stressful situation where escape is desired but obstructed, distinguishing it from hopelessness (Gilbert & Allan, 1998) since the individual may not have relinquished hope of being able to escape in the future.

An example of an entrapment event follows:

A woman is living in a room with her young son in a hostel. She is offered a better flat by a housing association. She accepts this, but it turns out to have

major structural defects (crumbling walls etc). The housing association de-
nies all responsibility and is not willing to undertake the work required. She
contacts a surveyor from Citizens Advice Bureau who is willing to initiate
legal proceedings given she is assured that the Housing Association has responsibility for the repairs. She has already given her notice at the hostel and
they have rented out the room she left. She has to move in with her estranged
partner's mother with whom she has a poor relationship. There is no sign
that the housing situation will be sorted out in the near future and she has to
remain in uncomfortable and inconvenient surroundings.

Entrapment in humans can either be external, wanting to escape from difficult
circumstances as described by the events above, or internal, wanting to escape
from negative thoughts or feelings (Gilbert & Allan, 1998). Much research has
focused on how defeat and entrapment may be factors in either the development
of various psychological disorders or in their maintenance such as depression
and PTSD although less evidence exists for a link between them in anxiety and
suicide (Taylor et al., 2011). Different studies have looked at whether these are
two different constructs are one and the same. Some argue that defeat and entrapment co-occur and set up a depressogenic loop – a person experiences a
defeat which leads to entrapment and further defeat leading to depression and
anxiety (Griffiths et al., 2014). There are those who argue that really these are
two facets of the same construct with each influencing the other (Taylor et al.,
2011) as shown from factor analyses on both the Defeat and Entrapment scales
which are very highly correlated (Taylor, Gooding, Wood, & Tarrier, 2014). Conversely, other researchers have shown them to be separate constructs but highly
associated using more sophisticated statistical techniques (Forkmann, Teismann,
Stenzel, Glaesmer, & de Beurs, 2018).

As with the research on loss and humiliation, the studies above focus on the
individual's *perception* of defeat and entrapment by measuring common triggers
with the Defeat Scale and Entrapment Scale (Gilbert & Allan, 1998). They argue that the triggers for defeat and entrapment are not just external (e.g. life
events or other life stresses) but can also become internalised meaning the individuals responses to events are of feelings of humiliation, entrapment or defeat.
They argue that it is the *perceptions* related to defeat and entrapment that are
centrally important. A meta-analysis of perceptions of defeat and entrapment
and their relationship to depression, anxiety, suicide and PTSD (Siddaway
et al., 2015) analysed 40 studies and found strong effect sizes (around $r = 0.60$)
which were similar in size across all four psychiatric disorders with defeat particularly strong in depression ($r = 0.73$). Similar-sized relationships across four
different psychiatric disorders suggest that perceptions of defeat and entrapment
are trans-diagnostic constructs. However, for many, the perceptions of defeat
and entrapment will come from the situation in which they find themselves.
Whilst for some, the lack of assertiveness and practical coping skills, together
with pessimism, may lead to an acceptance of entrapment where solutions are
in fact available, the inactivity itself may lead to a worsening of the entrapping

situation. Thus, a focus on the internal state alone is likely to miss the external constraints which exist.

The concept of D-matching events was further developed by the Bedford Square team to involve the concept of entrapment. This entrapping aspect involves an event where an individual is unable to escape or is effectively imprisoned to some degree by the preceding chronic difficulty – reminiscent of the literature on animal studies. In their sample, Brown and colleagues found that people experiencing events which were rated as having a high degree of entrapment (or humiliation) and loss were three times more likely to become depressed compared to those experiencing events which were only rated as involving loss (see the earlier figure) (Brown et al., 1995). Humiliation and entrapment were not significantly correlated suggesting two independent constructs. Kendler and colleagues did not find entrapment events to be predictive of an onset of depression, but significantly predictive of mixed depression and anxiety (Kendler et al., 2003).

Commitments, disappointments and goal frustration

Finally, another type of personalised severe event is one that matches a prior area of high commitment. This requires evidence of prior planful behaviour and investment to achieve particular positive goals (e.g. sustained effort in study involving some sacrifice to achieve a good degree) or investing in a role (e.g. becoming a parent and giving up a favoured job to focus on childcare). This is subsequently followed by an event that has a negative impact in the context of the prior investment or commitment. Thus, the categorisation of a C-matching severe event involves disappointment in the area of commitment. For example, failing a professional exam after months of hard work and dedication to study and practice; failing to become pregnant following a first IVF trial. What is unusual about these severe life events compared to the D-matching events described above is that the prior conditions can be positive and involve positive coping and high functioning. The event then becomes an unexpected blow to a sense of achievement.

In the Islington study (study 3 in Appendix 1), Brown and colleagues measured commitment levels in key roles a year prior to the investigation of the following life events and onset of depression (Brown, Bifulco, & Harris, 1987). This ensured that the rating of commitment was not influenced by the event itself thus leading to an exaggerated view of the prior commitment. However, it could also be rated in cross-sectional or retrospective study by collecting behavioural evidence of such commitment. Analysis showed that 31% of the 130 community women studied prospectively having a matching C-event, and of these, 40% had new onsets of depression compared with 14% without a C-event (p < 0.01) (Brown et al., 1987). The two types of matching events (C and D) were found to be uncorrelated. These findings revealed the utility of both of the dimensions of commitment and difficulties as important longstanding contextual factors that interplay with current life events in the aetiology of disorder.

The following pregnancy examples illustrate both loss and matching events, with the second example also having other characteristics of the dimensions discussed in this chapter. This indicates that for complex events that happen in life, several damaging characteristics can be present and influential.

Example of pregnancy severe events with matching difficulties

Sarah and her partner have been trying to get pregnant for two years and are offered a round of IVF. The treatment is unsuccessful, but the doctors say that there is some chance they may succeed in the future if they continue. This has an impact on the area of identity (as a parent) and achievement (not being able to reach goal of having a child). It is also a loss for Sarah and her partner (of cherished idea) as they have been unsuccessful in conceiving despite going through IVF with potentially high hopes. [Loss event; **D matching event; C-matching event**.]

Veronica and her partner have not been able to have a baby for five years. She has undergone numerous medical procedures and rounds of IVF treatment which have not been successful. She has undergone another procedure which was initially successful but ended in a miscarriage. They have now been told that it is very unlikely that she will be able to carry a pregnancy. Veronica's ethnic background and community values mean that being childless carries stigma for women. This event has an impact on her identity as a parent and achievement in reaching the goal of having a baby. It also features loss, but with an element of 'entrapment', in that the elements of 'escape' have been blocked, and there is more of a sense of finality to their situation. Given the stigmatising element in Veronica's cultural background, it also has aspects of humiliation. [**Loss event, C-matching event; D-matching event with entrapment; Humiliation event**.]

A new model of event-related need (ASIA)

Understanding the link between types of severe life events and a depression response calls into question what it is about a person's psychological state that is threatened, challenged or changed by the event. This would help explain why the events are upsetting and why some can become overwhelming. It can also help with making ratings of severe life events as we consider what aspects of an event could be viewed as threatening to the individual.

For this reason, we have constructed the conceptual needs model of ASIA as briefly outlined in the introduction. We have taken key elements from both Maslow and Beck in determining four basic psychological needs which we believe are threatened by severe life events. From Beck's cognitive triad, we took negative perception of the Future (Achievement); the World (Security); the Self (Identity); to which was added People (Attachment). This also utilises Maslow's hierarchy of needs, not including the physiological level or the uppermost self-actualisation. We will describe each in turn.

Attachment – being loved

Since Bowlby, the theory and concept of attachment has received wide-ranging attention in both the research and clinical fields (Bowlby, 1980). He identified attachment to close others as a basic need that in childhood determines our ability to form close bonds with others and a belief in a positive and responsive social environment. A key element is trust of others, and this is carried forward as part of the internal working model which forms the characteristic view of others. When distorted, mistrust, as well as fear of rejection, fear of abandonment and anger are readily triggered by social interactions. These persist in to adulthood with attachment figures including partners, parents, siblings and close confidants. The result is the formation of adult relationships that prove unsupportive and accompanied by interpersonal life events around 'making and breaking of affectional bonds' (Bowlby, 1979).

Life events which impact on the area of attachment involve some degree of change in a relationship with someone with whom an individual has close ties, usually a partner, parent, child or confidant. When these events are severe, they involve a negative change in a relationship which could involve loss of the person or loss of the positive relationship, for example, through rejection, humiliation or interpersonal conflict. Loss may be common, for example, separation from partner. Other events involving rejection or humiliation (learns of partner's affair, confidant spreading malicious rumours) can also be destructive of attachment needs and disturb the individual's sense of trust.

Security – being safe

A need for security in relation to safety and the environment is necessary for normal functioning. Where people have fears of the outside world, for example a heightened sense of crime and danger in the streets, this can impede their daily life. We need to feel that the world is predictable and essentially benign in order to undertake basic daily actions. The concept is also utilised in Attachment Theory with security being a basic developmental requirement for both physical and psychological health in childhood (Bowlby, 1988). Maslow placed 'safety' in his hierarchy as being the second most important determinant of human motivation after physiological needs (Maslow, 1971).

Many of the severe life events we had studied were related to physical safety with threat linked to uncertainty around routines or physical danger or through health events. (See also trauma events described in the next chapter.) Examples could be on a national/community level such as war, earthquake, terror attacks or an individual level such as a car crash or diagnosis of cancer. There is often an erosion of the 'world as being a safe place' as these events shake an individual's concept of the safety and certainty around them. Danger events outlined earlier in the chapter would constitute threats to actual security and feelings of security. These can denote future losses (e.g. diagnosis of cancer) but can also encompass other aspects of danger to the self or close others or to a predictable future.

Identity – self-esteem and belonging

Early research undertaken on identity recognised its dual psychological and social aspects, and it is defined as the 'personal meaning people ascribe to the multiple social categories to which they claim membership' (Deaux, 1993) (Abstract). As such, it covers both subjective and objective social experience. It involves belonging to a valued group as well as feeling worthy as a person. Psychological analysis has typically focused on the influence of social context on self-esteem, exploring how individuals organise their qualities or traits and how these apply to the self across situations and in relation to poor mental health (Mann, Hosman, Schaalma, & De Vries, 2004).

Sociological approaches from the 1960s (McCall & Simmons, 1966) invoke social roles as the basis of identity (as student, worker, partner, parent, community leader), and the variety of roles present is often taken as a marker of health. The hierarchy of role identities is considered to be related to their value. These increase perceptions of self-worth of belonging and positive identity. Both single and multiple aspects of self-identity are conceptually relevant with a central core tied to life-narrative, personal memory and consistency across situations juxtaposed with selves expressed differently according to role and situation demands (Kang, Shaver, Sue, Min, & Jing, 2003). The post-modern 'protean' self is one which it is argued transforms as situations require (Brown, Dutton, & Cook, 2001). This is seen to increase adaptability to the change required in the modern world. Thus, younger individuals are seen to have more superficial attachment to roles and increased adaptability to change, whereas individuals from earlier generations form more singular attachment to limited roles with duty mitigating against increased change. Such differences in identity formation have implications for role-performance, relationship stability, attachment style and adaptation to loss. This in turn will differentially affect self-esteem, wellbeing and mental health.

The types of roles investigated in risk for psychological disorder research involve those potentially related to lower social status, for example, female gender, social exclusion, minority ethnic status or LGBTQ status (NATCEN, edited by O'Connor & Nazroo, 2002). For example, there are psychological concerns over why female identities persist in being associated with low self-esteem and related emotional disorders and sociological concerns over why many women feel trapped and unrewarded by their roles (Nolen-Hoeksema et al., 1999). Social exclusion is defined as 'when individuals or areas suffer from a combination of linked problems such as unemployment, poor skills, low incomes, poor housing, high crime environments, bad health and family breakdown' (Millar, 2007). This is extended to those 'socially isolated … with weak social relatedness' (Peace, 2001). This broad definition invokes a range of psychosocial ill-effects including: 'psychological problems, relationship problems, loss of identity, loss of cultural affiliations, de-structuring of the person, loss of purpose, de-integration from family ties, …and de-integration from social relations' (op cit). Women who have fallen outside social 'safety nets' include single parents, those excluded from employment opportunities, those lacking economic independence, those victimised by violence, those failing to access services and those constrained by cultural/ethnic traditions. Despite increases in women's opportunities and participation over the last 30 years, there are increasing numbers of women with such experience.

However, there are aspects of identity disturbance, which may emanate from sources other than isolation – due to the burden of numerous roles and the role strain resulting (Brown, Bifulco, Veiel, & Andrews, 1990). Here, despite the presence of alternatives, individuals are constrained by stressors, burdens and entrapment within their roles. Many women are restricted by caring roles, whether of young children and families or of elderly relatives, and strained by life events and difficulties in roles/relationships which limit any reward potential. Some will be prey to humiliation events involving public rejections or belittling which casts doubt on the value of the role. Life events may also involve loss of role or relationship which can damage a sense of identity. Both the range and quality of roles need to be rewarding to confer wellbeing. Events related to identity also involve failure of belonging, stigma and loss of social status. This includes humiliation events involving 'put downs' and stigma associated with antisocial actions of close others.

Achievement – having success

Having success in life, and having personal goals to reach, is a basic psychological need. This can include those work and career-related (working towards a promotion, getting a new job, getting a first job), study-related (getting required results and qualifications) or relating to reproduction (conceiving, having a baby) or also skill-based (e.g. learning to drive, playing the piano). In different cultures, perceptions of worthy goals may vary, with some goals being of great importance in some cultures but not in others – such as marriage, financial success and educational attainment. In the psychological literature, a distinction has been made between mastery goals which involve competence and achievement goals which relate to social acknowledgement of success (Elliot & Hulleman, 2017). The mastery goals are thought to be associated with a positive cognitive outlook, whilst the achievement goals focus more on social comparisons. With negative distortion of cognitions, this can lead to unrealistic goals being set, or denigration of personal success, or the belief that others will always achieve more.

Life events which impact negatively on the realm of achievement have been defined as 'events that prevented, thwarted or hindered an individual reaching a goal' (Abela, 2002). These usually involve failure in an area of prior high commitment with directed activity whether in education, work or key roles. These of course will vary and can include goals such as trying to get pregnant as well as getting a promotion or passing an exam. A critical element is evidence of prior goal-directed activity which would link to a sense of achievement if the goal was realised. Goal frustration events are those most likely to impinge on achievement needs. These events involve disappointment in a worked-for goal. Examples such as failure to become pregnant during expensive IVF treatment would be included due to the commitment to the desired goal. This would include the pre-viously outlined concepts of C-events (matching areas of commitment) and those labelled as goal frustration. Research has found that commitment to an area of life has also been linked to gender differences in the experiences of life events which precede an onset of depression when looking at more traditional male and female roles (Kendler, Thornton, & Prescott, 2001). It was found that men responded more to severe life events around work and financial disappointments than women who were more focused on attachment needs. This was echoed in the couples study utilising the LEDS whereby even when experiencing a joint severe event those involving children affected the female partners significantly more (Nazroo et al., 1997). Furthermore, unemployment has been found to be particularly related to disorder in men and has been labelled as a type of goal frustration (Eales, 1988). A study of men soon after being made unemployed showed 14% developed depression following job loss over the first six months of unemployment. An increased risk of onset was associated with three factors: lack of an intimate relationship with a wife or girlfriend, trait shyness and pre-existing economic difficulties (op cit).

A study of life events in relation to physical illness (abdominal pain patients at a gastrointestinal clinic) was conducted using the LEDS with the new category of goal frustration tested (Craig & Brown, 1994). Three groups included patients with organic illness (e.g. ulcerative colitis or pancreatitis) those with functional problems (e.g. dyspepsia or irritable bowel syndrome) and healthy controls. Find-ings showed double the rate of severe events involving goal frustration in the organic group (54%) compared to a functional group (24%) and with only 9% in a healthy comparison group in the 36 weeks before onset.

Events relating to achievement are also considered to relate to personality characteristics. For example, using Beck's Sociotropy/Autonomy Scale, it was recorded that onset or exacerbation of depression symptoms occur for sociotropic individuals experiencing more negative interpersonal events than achievement events and for autonomous-achievement patients experiencing more achieve-ment events than interpersonal events (Hammen, Ellicott, Gitlin, & Jamison, 1989). The various needs outlined can thus be seen to overlap – with identity wrapped up in our attachments and achievements, security both material but also found in reciprocal relationships which can make us feel safe, achievement can involve goals that increase security, etc.

Figure 2.6 gives a graphic representative of the needs and types of severe life events.

A model for clinical practice

Above we have highlighted how characteristics of severe life events can be related to the four areas of need to explain the emotional impact of events on individuals. An individual could experience a loss in attachment (relationship breakup); secu-rity (house fire/loss of possessions); identity (inability to conceive) or achievement (not getting a promotion). It is likely that there may be more than one dimension

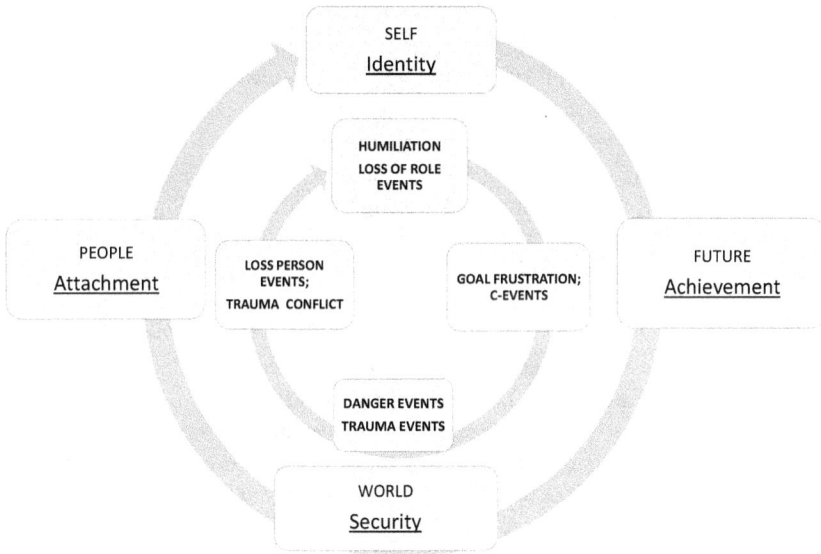

Figure 2.6 ASIA needs and related severe events.

at play in certain life events with the more damaging events impacting on more than one dimension and area of need. One reason that humiliation events are particularly potent for depression is that they often involve aspects of attachment, security and identity damage. For example, a rejecting separation by partner could involve both attachment and security loss. A close family member being imprisoned for violent crime could invoke both security and identity in relation to social status in the community. The link between psychological need and type of severe life event is further explained in terms of vulnerability and will be outlined in Chapter 4. Thus, factors identified as predisposing individuals to depression include insecure attachment style (Bifulco, Moran, Ball, & Bernazzani, 2002), low self-esteem (Brown, Bifulco, Veiel, Andrews, 1990), helplessness (Harris, Brown, & Bifulco, 1990) and lower social status including gender (Bebbington, Dean, Der, Hurry, & et al., 1991). These all have implications for the four-fold model and will be examined in Chapter 4.

At the start of therapeutic intervention, a longitudinal formulation of client difficulties includes an understanding of the clients' early life experiences and the beliefs about themselves, others and world around them and how the life event that precipitated the problem then re-activates the underlying beliefs that the client has formed leading to their current state of psychological disorder. Such models are used in disorder-specific formulations such as depression and anxiety disorders or in a less diagnostic sense to develop an understanding of why the particular client has presented at this particular time. Clinical formulation has been applied across different specific models (Dallos & Johnstone, 2014) or for use in an integrative model such as the '5 P's' approach which looks at the **P**resenting problem, that the client comes with; **P**redisposing factors, childhood or distal factors; **P**recipitating event, what event they link their problem to; **P**erpetuating factors that maintains the problem and **P**rotective factors involving skills and assets to overcome the problem (Dudley & Kuyken, 2006). Both the 5 P's and CBT formulations are critically interested in how the precipitating life event fits within the individual's earlier experience, perceptions and expectations.

In clinical work, the precipitating event may be described in minimal detail whereas the different aspects of the 5 P's model are more fully explored with more weight given to different areas depending on the therapeutic model. In a classical CBT formulation and therapy, more time may be spent on the current perpetuating factors, that is, those ongoing difficulties together with ineffective coping behaviours. Sometimes, it is quite clear why a certain life event may have led to the current functioning problem, but at other times, it is not so obvious. Having a more comprehensive assessment of the events themselves – by looking at the context and dimensions described above could give a more complex understanding of what a particular life event threatened in leading to the current symptomatology. This approach could help the clinician understand why a particular severe life event had such a far-reaching effect on an individual and why it might have provoked, for example, anxiety rather than depression. An individual who experienced a humiliating work event (threat to self-esteem and achievement) may then be encouraged to explore her needs in terms of expectations and self-identity which may in turn relate to early life experience. Through exploring the different features of events, we are offering up meaning to both clinician and client.

Notes

1 See contacts on lifespantraining.org.uk
2 An odds ratio (OR) is a statistic that quantifies the strength of the association between two events or effect size. The OR represents the odds that an outcome will occur given a particular exposure compared to the odds of the outcome occurring in the absence of that exposure. An odds ratio of one implies that the event is equally likely in both groups. An odds ratio greater than one implies that the event is more likely in the first group.

3   Trauma – extreme life events

The previous chapter examined features of severe life events to identify aspects which make them psychologically damaging, linked to challenges to basic needs. However, we have not so far discussed trauma events, which deserve additional discussion for two reasons. First, trauma events are a necessary diagnostic element of Post-Traumatic Stress Disorder (PTSD), and therefore their definition is critical to this diagnosis, so understanding how these are correctly classified is important in clinical contexts. Second, trauma events are among the most intense types of life events and can lead to longer-lasting vulnerability for an individual. This is particularly true when the trauma experience occurs in childhood or adolescence and can cause developmental harms which impact later in life. However, certain adult trauma experience can also have this effect including domestic violence, rape or war experience, setting up longer-term psychological damage. Therefore, trauma events are here considered as a separate category of life event.

Trauma has a double-edged meaning. On the one hand, it refers to trauma exposure which fits the category of an extreme type of life event (or longer-term problem) as discussed in pervious chapters. On the other hand, it can refer to the impact of trauma (i.e. being traumatised), and this can have specific characteristics which can extend further than depression to include traumatic stress responses. Within PTSD definitions, these involve damaged processing of the life-threatening event, for example, problems with remembering (over-remembering or amnesia) for the event as well as other emotional, cognitive and physical responses which lead to either constant vigilance or a shutdown of emotions. Such events are critical to PTSD diagnosis where the event (labelled as Criterion A) is a necessary feature (DSM–5) (APA, 2013):

Criterion A in PTSD describes trauma exposure thus:

The person is exposed to death, threatened death, actual or threatened serious injury, or actual or threatened sexual violence, in the following way(s):

- Direct exposure
- Witnessing the trauma
- Learning that a relative or close friend was exposed to a trauma
- Indirect exposure to aversive details of the trauma, usually in the course of professional duties (e.g. first responders, medics).

Trauma events are therefore an extreme type of life event which inherently involves danger to life. However, it can also include witnessing such dangerous events or indeed learning of them from a close relative or friend and experiencing them second hand. It also includes experiences of emergency services who witness such trauma in their professional capacity (Fjeldheim et al., 2014). The prevalence of trauma events is therefore widened by such witnessing or professional involvement with other people's trauma experience.

Trauma events are expected to cause psychological 'wounding' to the individual experiencing them. They convey that the world is a dangerous and damaging place, and these experiences can undermine belief in a settled and happy future. Trauma events can pose particular barriers to processing of information and emotion involved in the impact. Memory of the event can invoke terror and helplessness and 'inescapable shock' (van der Kolk, 2015):

> Even years later traumatized people often have enormous difficulty telling other people what happened to them. Their bodies reexperience terror, rage and helplessness, as well as the impulse to fight or flee, but these feelings are almost impossible to articulate. Trauma by nature drives us to the edge of comprehension, cutting us off from language based on common experience or an imaginable past. (van der Kolk, 2015) (p. 43)

PTSD as a clinical disorder includes four different criteria in addition to that of the trauma event. All need to be present for at least a month to qualify for a clinical rating. The response can involve intrusive thoughts of the trauma event such as flashbacks or nightmares. It can also include avoidance in terms of shutting off from thoughts or reminders of the event. There are also negative alterations in cognitions or mood including poor recall of the event or exaggerated sense of blame of self or towards others. Alterations in arousal or reactivity such as hypervigilance or destructive behaviour are included. In addition, certain other specifications can be met – dissociative response when the individual feels depersonalisation (detached from the self) or derealisation (feeling things are not real). Another specification is that all criteria are still met at least six months after the trauma event. Many if not most who experience trauma can show these symptoms immediately after the event, but the disorder is only classified if these continue for at least six months afterwards.

In his seminal book *The body keeps the score*, Bessel van der Kolk describes the somatic elements of trauma response (van der Kolk, 2015). He describes responses to danger in terms of three stages – at the first signs of danger, most of us socially engage by calling out for help or support. But if the danger is very immediate or there is no source of help, then we use flight or fight to survive. If this fails or we cannot escape due to entrapment, then psychologically and physically, we shut down and expend as little energy as possible in a state of freeze or collapse. This is considered the traumatised response. In physiological terms, the 'emergency system' in the dorsal vagal complex (DVC) is activated. The vagus nerve is the longest cranial nerve which runs all the way from the brain stem to part of the colon. Its functions involve somatic components, sensations felt on the skin or muscles and visceral components and sensations felt in the organs of the body. This system reaches to the stomach, kidneys and intestines and drastically reduces metabolism throughout the body. The heart rate plunges, there is difficulty breathing and the gut stops working or empties. This is the stage at which physical disengagement collapse and freeze occurs. Then, psychological awareness shuts down, and we may even fail to register physical pain. Such immobilisation is thus seen to be at the root of most trauma. Longer-term effects involve the loss of a sense of self, of agency and of feeling (van der Kolk, 2015).

Even though three-quarters of people will be exposed to trauma events at some point in their lives, only a small minority of people in the population develop PTSD. It is estimated that there is about 8% lifetime and 4% yearly prevalence in the population (Atwoli, Stein, Koenen, & McLaughlin, 2015). A large-scale WHO study examined the prevalence of trauma events and PTSD in 24 countries in 69,000 adults (Kessler et al., 2017). As many as 70% of the sample had experienced lifetime trauma events, with an average of three trauma events per person. There were seven categories of trauma events which included:

- War (e.g. combatant, civilian in war zone, relief worker, refugee);
- Physical violence (e.g. physically attacked, mugged);
- Intimate partner or sexual violence (raped, sexually assaulted, stalked, physically abused by a romantic partner);
- Accidents (toxic chemical spill, other man-made disaster, natural disaster, life-threatening motor vehicle collision, accident where the respondent caused serious injury to another person, life-threatening illness);
- Unexpected or traumatic death of a loved one;
- Traumas to other people (child had life-threatening illness, witnessed other trauma);
- 'Other' traumas.

Trauma events also include those in childhood, which is outside the remit of this chapter – see Chapter 4 for a discussion of childhood trauma. This is linked in some classifications to complex PTSD trauma diagnoses (van der Kolk, 2001). Trauma exposure involving interpersonal violence has the highest risk of PTSD. Experiences of rape (13%), other sexual assault (15%) and being stalked (10%) led to greatest risk of disorder (Kessler et al., 2017). A fifth category – unexpected death of a loved one (12%) – was a very common trauma but with low PTSD risk. The broad category of intimate partner sexual violence accounted for nearly 43% of all people per year developing PTSD.

The question therefore arises as to how to accurately identify trauma events, with these potentially extreme reactions occurring, and to determine whether they are different in nature from other severe life events. It will be argued here that they can be viewed as a particular extreme subset of life events with identifiable characteristics that can be measured alongside other types of life event. The research tells us that trauma events often occur in multiples and alongside other severe life events. Just how they relate to other types of severe life events and whether these events cluster around trauma may help us understand whether this can further psychologically disable a person (Jin, Sun, Wang, An, & Xu, 2018). Additionally, it is known even within the trauma categorisation that some trauma events are more likely to provoke PTSD than others (Carmassi et al., 2014). Additionally, some negative life events that fall short of current trauma definitions, such as certain instances of infidelity and relationship disturbances, can also relate to PTSD (Gold, Marx, Soler-Baillo, & Sloan, 2005). It appears that further explication of trauma events is helpful to better understand how trauma events occur and the impact they might have.

Despite its relative infrequency, PTSD is associated with some of the widest use of health care systems and a high associated cost per patient. Thus, an understanding of responses to trauma events in relation to preventative work is important (Boscarino, 2004; Kessler, 2000). Traumatic events can occur within a context of other negative experiences such as ongoing deprivation or substance abuse which also may give clues to added stress burden or dose effects (Kim, Ford, Howard, & Bradford, 2010). Given severe life events tend to cluster within the same individuals (Bifulco, Brown, Moran, Ball, & Campbell, 1998; Foley, Neale, & Kendler, 1996; Kendler, Neale, Kessler, Heath, & Eaves, 1993), this may help to explain why PTSD frequently co-occurs with other psychiatric diagnoses (Contractor et al., 2014; Grubaugh, Long, Elhai, Frueh, & Magruder, 2010) as well as explaining why events that do not meet PTSD criterion can be related to PTSD (Bodkin, Pope, Detke, & Hudson, 2007; Van Hooff, McFarlane, Baur, Abraham, & Barnes, 2009). This is borne out by research which illustrates that experiencing a severe negative life event can add to the impact of trauma experience (Brewin, Andrews, & Valentine, 2000).

Another issue concerns timing and longer-term harm imposed by trauma events. Studies show that delayed PTSD onset is often associated with experiencing severe life events, sometimes many years after the initial trauma (Andrews, Brewin, Rose, & Kirk, 2000; Boscarino & Adams, 2009; Horesh, Solomon, Zerach, & Ein-Dor, 2011). Additionally, PTSD symptomatology increases after experiencing a subsequent severe life event or trauma (Schock, Böttche, Rosner, Wenk-Ansohn, & Knaevelsrud, 2016). This illustrates the importance for both clinicians and researchers to examine in detail not only the index trauma(s) but also any stressful experiences surrounding the trauma. Those who fail to assess the impact of other contextual factors might misattribute the cause of distress or ignore their intersecting effects which could further decrease resilience and increase the likelihood of disorder, greater symptomatology or co-occurring disorder. The concept of trauma will now be linked to the dimensions of events covered in Chapter 2.

Possible dimensions of trauma events

The characteristics of severe events outlined in the previous chapter will be examined to see if they can also be applied to trauma events. Clearly, trauma events invoke notions of danger and extreme threats to security by definition, given they threaten death, injury or assault. This can lead to individuals having to overhaul their previous beliefs, with cognitive restructuring around concepts of safety and self-assessment (Brewin, 2014). Obvious examples are those with PTSD symptoms risk who live with danger on a day-to-day basis, including war combatants, victims of stalking or victims of natural disasters (Kessler et al., 2017; Norris & Slone, 2013; Xu & Liao, 2011). The perception of life threat is significantly associated with PTSD (Larsen & Berenbaum, 2017), even after adjusting for specific trauma events (Heir, Blix, & Knatten, 2016).

Loss has already been defined in broad terms (e.g. loss of person, home or of a cherished idea), with the permanence of such loss denoting higher severity ratings and with bereavement having particular impact. Most definitions of trauma include losses of close others by either sudden or violent death, and this is commonly associated with PTSD symptoms in the general population (O'Connor, 2010). In addition, serious injury and sexual assault may involve aspects of loss, for example, through loss of role whereby an accidental injury prevents the individual working, or loss of sexual functioning after rape with damage to a partner relationship. Studies show that events involving emotional loss are significantly associated with PTSD symptoms above and beyond the standard event Criterion-A stressors (Carlson, Smith, & Dalenberg, 2013). This indicates that loss may be a central aspect of certain trauma events (O'Connor, 2010). This may occur even when such bereavements are non-violent, but when involving sudden or untimely elements such as the death of a child from accident or chronic illness.

As outlined earlier, feelings of anger, shame and guilt are often associated with trauma impact, and humiliation may underlie some of the association between traumatic events and PTSD (Lee, Scragg, & Turner, 2001). Shame and anger often follow a violent event and raise PTSD risk (Andrews et al., 2000). Other research suggests that the negative social impact of public humiliation, ridicule or rejection can be experienced as more distressing than the more standard trauma events (Carleton, Peluso, Collimore, & Asmundson, 2011) and can lead to PTSD symptoms (Erwin, Heimberg, Marx, & Franklin, 2006; Guðmundsdóttir, 2016). In particular, persistent humiliation can lead to significantly lower psychological functioning than periodic exposure to violence (Barber, McNeely, Olsen, Belli, & Doty, 2016).

Entrapment has also been identified as a feature of trauma events which can lead to a shutdown in physiological systems when escape is impossible (Griffiths, Wood, Maltby, Taylor, & Tai, 2014). Entrapping trauma events are also strongly related to suicidal behaviour in those with PTSD (Panagioti, Gooding, Taylor, & Tarrier, 2012). Extreme entrapping trauma situations can involve torture and hostage situations, but more common domestic abuse can also feature entrapment when powerful partners curtail victims' access to resources and supportive others. Other types of entrapment can follow from burdensome caring experience (van den Born-van Zanten, Dongelmans, Dettling-Ihnenfeldt, Vink, & van der Schaaf, 2016) including parents caring for children with chronic illnesses (Cabizuca, Marques-Portella, Mendlowicz, Coutinho, & Figueira, 2009).

Similar effects are found in victims of school and workplace bullying and terrorising who find they can't readily escape (Nielsen, Tangen, Idsoe, Matthiesen, & Magerøy, 2015).

Whilst trauma can be argued to be a subset of severe life events, is it the case that all trauma events would always qualify as severe events? Surprisingly, not all do. This is because trauma events can have initial impact from the day they occur. However, severe events require at least two weeks continuous exposure for full impact to develop likely life changes. Thus, some events might be traumatic in the short term (e.g. seeing a horrific street accident to a stranger) but ultimately prove not to have longer-term effect on the individual's life going forward. An example occurred during our own CLEAR research project which highlights the differentiation. A young man was travelling for a gap year alone. He went to Thailand and was there when the tsunami occurred. However, he was swiftly evacuated by the British Embassy with other Britons, and although he did witness some of the devastation in the countryside and thinks he may have seen some dead bodies, he lost nobody close to him nor his home or possessions and was himself unhurt. By the end of two weeks, he was safe at home in the UK, so whilst the event of being in the tsunami had the highest threat in the short term ('marked'), longer term this reduced to only 'some' threat. Yet this could constitute a trauma event due to the shocking and unexpected catastrophe and potential threat to life and witnessing others threat to life. In fact, it did not in fact make any fundamental difference to his own life.

Overlap of severe events and trauma events

Whilst the Bedford Square team did not specifically publish on trauma life events, in order to examine how attributes of severe events may overlap with trauma classifications, a secondary analysis of published LEDS event data was more recently undertaken (Spence, Kagan, & Bifulco, 2019). This was data from a London community sample of 110 vulnerable women seen prospectively (Coping study 5 – see Appendix 1) (Bifulco et al., 1998). Across all respondents, the LEDS interview had classified 1,232 separate life events in an 18-month period. The reanalysis aim was to re-examine those cases with the most 'marked' threat ratings as potential candidates for a scoring of trauma events. A post hoc analysis applied a checklist of traumatic events, the Life Events Checklist for DSM-5 (LEC-5) (Weathers et al., 2013). This is a standardised questionnaire which outlines 17 different categories of trauma events – see Figure 3.1. (It should be noted that PTSD was not assessed in this study.)

The researchers applied these items to the summarised events (inter-rater reliability between independent ratings proved to be $\kappa = 0.90$) and found 4% of events meeting Criterion-A Trauma across 40 respondents. Most involved physical assault (39%) or death/life threatening illness (28%). There were fewer sexual assaults (11%), accidents (13%) or severe human suffering (9% e.g. suicide attempt of other, stillbirth). Analysis showed that of those individuals who were categorised as having experienced an LEC-5 trauma event, most (88%) had

- 1. Natural disaster (for example, flood, hurricane, tornado, earthquake)

- 2. Fire or explosion

- 3. Transportation accident (for example, car accident, boat accident, train wreck, plane crash)

- 4. Serious accident at work, home, or during recreational activity

- 5. Exposure to toxic substance (for example, dangerous chemicals, radiation)

- 6. Physical assault (for example, being attacked, hit, slapped, kicked, beaten up)

- 7. Assault with a weapon (for example, being shot, stabbed, threatened with a knife, gun, bomb)

- 8. Sexual assault (rape, attempted rape, made to perform any type of sexual act through force or threat of harm)

- 9. Other unwanted or uncomfortable sexual experience

- 10. Combat or exposure to a war-zone (in the military or as a civilian)

- 11. Captivity (for example, being kidnapped, abducted, held hostage, prisoner of war)

- 12. Life-threatening illness or injury

- 13. Severe human suffering

- 14. Sudden violent death (for example, homicide, suicide)

- 15. Sudden accidental death

- 16. Serious injury, harm, or death you caused to someone else

- 17. Any other very stressful event or experience

Figure 3.1 Questionnaire (LEC-5) of trauma events.

also experienced at least one other severe event as identified in the LEDS. Thus, trauma events and severe life events co-occurred in the same respondents.

The overlap of 'markedly' severe life events and LEC-5 trauma events was further examined to look for differences. This yielded 60 events across 22 respondents. There was only modest agreement between scorings of trauma versus a markedly severe event score ($\kappa = 0.36$, p < 0.0001). The LEDS 'marked threat' rating had a specificity of 97% (i.e. a true positive rate where trauma events were correctly identified) but a sensitivity of only 41% (i.e. a true negative rate where non-trauma events were correctly identified) with the trauma classification. The two measures are thus overlapping but by no means identical, suggesting that although trauma is likely to be an example of an event with marked threat, the concept of marked threat is broader than purely trauma. Thus, the shocking, often violent, threat to life aspects of trauma can of course constitute severe events, but other aspects of severity include for example being humiliated, losing someone, less extreme types of danger, and threats to other basic psychological needs.

The examination of pre-rated severe event dimensions (i.e. loss, danger, humiliation, entrapment) and the new trauma ratings (LEC-5) for this group of 'marked' threat events is shown in Figure 3.2. Nearly, all those events classified as trauma were scored additionally as having danger or loss with a further two categorised as having elements of humiliation. For non-trauma events, there was a wider spread of classifications including humiliation and entrapment. This latter category included events such as disability and death (e.g. serious chronic and potentially fatal illness of child or sudden, untimely but nonviolent death of close other); relationship crisis (14-year-old daughter ran away after a row and went missing in London); crime/legal (individual arrested for murder); material/housing (individual made homeless and was literally on the streets) and body image (disfigurement following illness).

% trauma events (Criterion A) with event feature

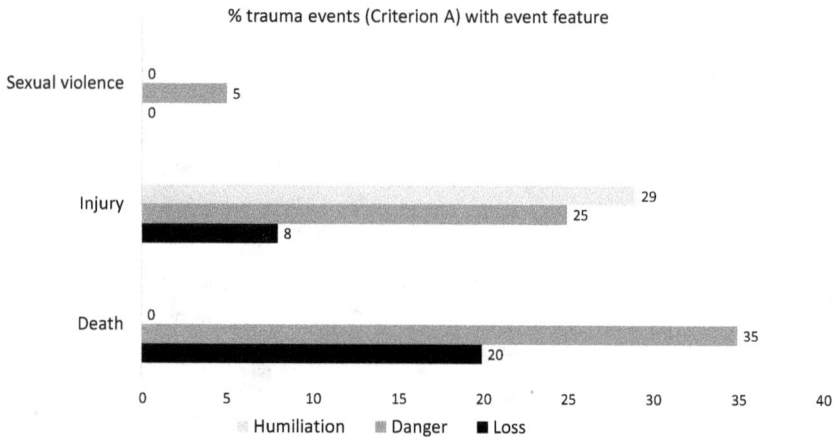

Figure 3.2 Overlap of trauma and marked severity ratings of life events.

Figure 3.2A shows that danger is rated in all three categories (sexual violence, injury or death) and thus a common characteristic of all types of trauma event, but is highest for the death category (35%) and then the injury category (25%). Humiliation was also high for the injury category (29%) but not the others. Loss was highest for the death category as expected (20%) but also occurred in the injury category (8%). Entrapment was not rated in any category.

In this next figure, the proportions of markedly threatening events where no trauma was rated are shown.

When events rated 'marked' on threat but not on trauma were examined it can be seen (Figure 3.3) that entrapment, humiliation, danger and loss were all rated as attributes. Humiliation in particular was high for both crime and relationship crisis categories. Loss occurred in all categories but was also highest in relationship crises. Danger occurred in most categories and was the highest recorded attribute in material/finance. Entrapment was the least common occurring in the body image, material/finance and disability/death categories at low levels.

Example of non-trauma, markedly severe event

The following description involves a case description of trauma and markedly severe event overlaps. It is an account of murder charges that one of the women in this sample experienced. This provides an interesting example where a 'markedly' threatening event did *not* constitute trauma according to the questionnaire criteria, but was nevertheless shocking and upsetting. The event occurred for a woman (Martha) whose sister Debby had a criminal record and was a drug-taker. Debby's partner was found dead, and a police investigation eventually charged her, but also implicated Martha, her brother and parents. Subsequently, Martha was arrested and was only released after 72 hours. The police

% with event feature

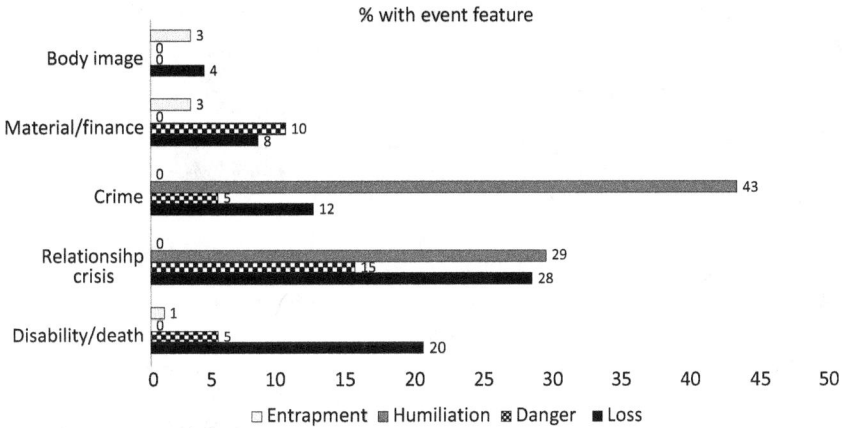

Figure 3.3 'Marked' threat events with no trauma, featuring the different event characteristics.

did not press charges. However, it later emerged that her brother Richard was in fact involved in the murder, and it was his confused confession that had implicated Debby as well as Martha herself. Richard then made a suicide attempt but survived. Although Martha was not charged, Debby was arrested for perverting the course of justice for withholding information, which carries a 12-year sentence, and Richard was charged with murder. Martha had to stand surety for her sister's bail for £15,000, and Debby had to live with her as a condition of her release. A further complication was that Debby had just given birth to her youngest child. The severe events identified here merited many 'marked' threat ratings and show features of humiliation (stigma from family 'delinquency') and danger throughout. The brother's suicide attempt also may involve trauma, although Martha was not particularly close to him. Interestingly, being charged with murder by the police does not itself fit in with the standard definition of trauma since it does not involve injury or threat to life.

This brief analysis suggests that trauma events commonly occur with severe life events, are a subset of events with marked threat and similarly have characteristics of loss, danger and humiliation. Thus, there is already some support for the further specification of the trauma concept for PTSD along potential dimensions already used for severe life events research. Potentially, adopting a dimensional approach to investigating what makes negative life events traumatic and what attributes are particularly traumatogenic would increase the range of experiences encompassed and also clarify the specific meaning of different subsets of trauma experience. Equally, this more qualitative or 'meaning' approach to understanding trauma would allow for a more considered approach when formulating treatment. It seeks to place the individual within their life context at the time of the event and also encompasses other related stressful events which impinge on the individual that may additional important therapeutic implications for managing trauma (e.g. through loss of other close support figures).

The importance of current context

The research on trauma implies that for many individuals, traumatic events occur within a context of other negative experiences such as ongoing deprivation or substance abuse (Dong et al., 2004; Dube et al., 2001; Hamel & Pampalon, 2002; Kim et al., 2010). Moreover, severe life events tend to cluster within the same individuals (Bifulco et al., 1998; Foley et al., 1996; Kendler, Neale, Kessler, Heath, & et al., 1993). Sarah's story, outlined below, illustrates how severe or traumatic events and ongoing problems can be related and cluster within the same individual's experiences. The trauma events occurring to this woman centred around domestic violence and attacks from her husband. This was also linked to other problems in his behaviour which led to financial, housing and legal difficulties. In fact, Sarah had the maximum number of life events, many severe, in our projects during an 18-month period because of her particularly complicated circumstances. Features of humiliation, entrapment, loss and danger can all be found in this account.

Example – Sarah's marital trauma

Sarah is a 35-year-old Scottish woman living in London in crowded conditions in a run-down council flat with her husband Steve and children. She works fulltime as a senior personal assistant in marketing but has had to start working evening shifts because she had problems finding a suitable child minder for her baby son. Her 34-year-old husband Steve is a television engineer who started his own business 18 months ago. This has put a financial strain on the household. Steve needs to be able to drive for his work but was banned from driving for a year after being caught drink-driving. Despite this, he carried on drink-driving and he was once again caught; this time, he was banned for two years, fined £400 and required to see a probation officer fortnightly.

Steve has become violent towards Sarah and frequently beats her up very badly. On each occasion, he has been drinking and taking drugs. When the attacks by Steve continue, giving her black eyes and causing her to lose two teeth, Sarah goes to the local police station where they have a special domestic violence unit. They tell her that she can prosecute her husband if she agrees and give her 24 hours in which to make up her mind. When she returns to the flat, she tells him what she has done. He once again becomes aggressive, and Sarah has to run next door to a neighbour who phones the police. The police arrive within minutes. Sarah decides she wants her husband to leave the flat, which he does, and hands his house keys over to her. However, later that evening, after the pub had shut, he turned up on the doorstep and Sarah let him return to the flat.

Steve's shop has been burgled five times in as many months, and to support the business, he has been using the flat rent money and therefore not paying the rent. Sarah did not realise this until she found a letter to him from the council and discovered that they were in rent arrears by £1,000. A few months later, Sarah received a summons letter from the council concerning non-payment of rent; she had believed that her husband had started repaying the rent and the rent arrears. However, the letter said that no rent had been paid and that they would now be evicted. In previous years, Sarah had taken out loans to clear her husband's debts. Sarah confronted Steve about the letter, and they argued, during which he became violent again and he hit her over the head with a coffee table. She made him leave the flat the next day and threw half of his clothes out on top of him from the balcony window. Steve went to stay with friends and has been telling people that she is mad, has spent all their money and that she is the problem. Sarah then explains her circumstances to the council, and they agree to delay – gave her a temporary eviction notice whereby if she defaults on one week's payment she will be evicted. Sarah also receives a visit from bailiffs for non-payment of bills, but the caretaker did not let them into the flat. Sarah phoned them and agreed to pay the outstanding amount on top of next year's bill. This is in addition to paying off rent arrears.

After she told Steve to leave, Sarah's friend told her that he had been sleeping with other women, and several days later, Steve tells Sarah that he has moved in with another women. Steve also comes back to the flat whilst Sarah is at work and takes everything of value, including the TV, stereo, her engagement ring and watch. He even takes pictures off the walls. Sarah gets legal advice about getting a court injunction but did not go ahead with it because of the cost. She also contacted her bank about their accounts and discovered Steve's business account is £5,000 overdrawn. After this, Sarah changes the locks. Steve later breaks down the door on more than one occasion when he is drunk, as he says he wants to see Sarah and their children.

Steve's business is burgled again, although Sarah suspects that this was set up by Steve in order to get the insurance money. Sarah wrote to the insurers to claim some of the money as maintenance for herself and the children. After this, Steve told the children that he would never see them again unless their mother dropped her claim on the money. Steve later gave up the business as it was in so much debt. He is now claiming benefits and very rarely gives Sarah money. She is also questioned by the police about Steve's whereabouts on a particular night. She lies to them but feels terrible afterwards when she is told that her husband's lock up next to his shop had been used to rape a woman. However, she still has not told the police the truth.

Sarah had a period of five weeks during which she didn't have any contact with Steve. Then, he phoned and visited, was repentant and wanted to see the children so she agreed to them going on holiday together with the children for two weeks. Whilst away, they had an argument and once again he became violent, leaving Sarah requiring hospital treatment and stitches. It was at this point Sarah had an onset of major depression. On their return, Steve took the car and also her camera. Sarah approached the council explaining the domestic violence situation, showed her stitches as proof, and they have made her a priority for re-housing on the basis of the violence.

Figure 3.4 shows summary ratings for Sarah's severe life events, with the violent attacks from her husband rated as trauma. However, it should be noted that many of her severe events have multiple other characteristics indicative of a range of serious events. It can be seen that many threatened her basic safety – not only the violence but also the possibility of being evicted and having nowhere for her and the children to live. There were also threats to attachment giving the length of their relationship and the betrayals involved. Also potentially to her self-identity given her pride in her career and prior family success.

i   *Financial difficulty scored 'moderate-low' starts after E8*
ii *Marital difficulty relationship scored 'marked' starts after E9*
iii *Numbered consecutively, although non-severe events not included*

Event No. Month	Summary of severe events- chronologically	Score on threat	Event attributes
E1 Jan	Husband's shop burgled 1st time	2-moderate	Loss
E2 Feb	Husband's shop burgled 2nd time	2-moderate	Loss
E3 Mar	Husband's shop burgled 3rd time	2-moderate	Loss
E4 Apr	Husband's shop burgled 4th time	2-moderate	Loss
E5 Apr	Husband stopped by police for drink/driving	2-moderate	Danger/ Humiliation
E6 Apr	Sarah discovers rent arrears	2-moderate	Danger/Humiliation
E7 Apr	Husband beats up Sarah and smashes up flat	1-marked	Danger/Humiliation/ **Trauma**
E8 Apr	Husband beats up Sarah again.	1-marked	Danger/Humiliation/**Trauma**
E9 Apr	Husband's shop burgled 5th time	2-moderate	Loss
E10 May	Husband reveals he has been taking drugs	2-moderate	Loss/Danger/Humiliation
E11 May	Husband in court re drink/driving – 1-year ban	2-moderate	Loss/Danger/Humiliation
E12 June	Husband caught drink/driving after ban	2-moderate	Danger/Humiliation
E13 Aug	She tell's mother-in-law she is going to police	2-moderate	Danger
E14 Aug	She reports husband's violence to the police	2-moderate	Danger

Figure 3.4 Sara's 30 severe life events in 20 months.

	New Year		
E15 April	Sarah finds summons from council due to arrears	2-moderate	Danger/ Humiliation
E16 April	Sarah gets beaten up by husband and throws him out	1-marked	Loss/Danger/Humiliation/ **Trauma** – D-event (6 months of marital difficulty)
E17 April	Friend tells Sarah that husband is 'screwing around' and seeing other women	1-marked	Loss/Danger/Humiliation – D-event (marital difficulty)
E18 April	Husband's shop burgled again – 6th time	2-moderate	Loss
E19 April	Husband returns and steals from flat	2-moderate	Loss/Danger/Humiliation – D-event
E20 April	Sarah seeks legal advice	2-moderate	Danger
E21 April	Husband tells her he is living with another woman	1-marked	Loss/Danger/Humiliation – D-event (marital difficulty)
E22 May	Husband breaks door down	2-moderate	Danger/Humiliation
E23 May	Husband gives up his business	2-moderate	Danger – D-event (financial difficulty)
E24 May	Husband breaks door down again	2-moderate	Danger/Humiliation – D-event (marital difficulty)
E25 May	Husband threatens not to see children again in reprisal for insurance money	2-moderate	Loss/Danger/Humiliation – D-event (marital difficulty)
E26 June	Son has been a bully at school	2-moderate	Loss/Humiliation
E27 June	Confidant doesn't answer Sarah's phone call – ends friendship	2-moderate	Loss/Danger/Humiliation
E28 Aug	Sarah questioned by police regarding husband's lock-up	2-moderate	Danger, D-event (financial difficulty)
E29 Aug **	Sarah holidays with husband & gets beaten up & needs stitches	1-marked	Danger/Humiliation/**Trauma**. D-event (marital difficulty)
E30 Aug	Husband refuses to return Sarah's car and camera	2-moderate	Loss/Danger – D-event (marital difficulty)

**onset major depression follows

Figure 3.4 Continued.

As Sarah's story helps to illustrate, the clustering of severe life events, their occurrence within the context of ongoing problems and their wearing effect on coping and support resources may help explain why PTSD is frequently comorbid with other psychiatric diagnoses (Contractor et al., 2014; Grubaugh et al., 2010) as well as why events that do not meet Criterion-A may be related to PTSD (Bodkin et al., 2007; Gold et al., 2005; Van Hooff et al., 2009). Indeed, severe events not reaching trauma criteria can still evoke a range of emotional reactions such as anger, sadness and anxiety as well as trigger negative cognitions around pessimism, self-doubt and hopelessness. This increase in general psychological distress can reduce an individual's available coping resources, which in turn may increase the likelihood of psychological disorder in general. Alternatively, a traumatic event may itself increase psychological distress reducing the ability to cope with other life events, further increasing distress and the likelihood of PTSD symptoms along with other disorder. Therefore, it should be unsurprising to conclude that the co-occurrence of severe events with present or past trauma(s) could be important for both PTSD and comorbid (co-occurring) disorder.

This illustrates the importance for clinicians and researchers to examine in detail not only the index trauma(s) but also any stressful experiences surrounding the trauma. Those who fail to assess the impact of other contextual factors might misattribute the cause of distress or ignore their intersecting effects which could be decreasing resilience and increasing the likelihood of disorder, greater symptomatology or comorbidity. This applies not just to proximal stressors but at times to those that have occurred across the lifespan, including childhood maltreatment.

It can be seen that many of Sarah's problems arise from her partner's antisocial behaviour. This seems to have been triggered by his business failures. However, it is noticeable that Sarah continued to let him visit after she threw him out and agreed to go on holiday with him at the end of the period. This speaks to her potential vulnerable attachment, in that she perhaps underestimates the danger from him and allows him second chances. Sarah's vulnerability will be examined in the next chapter. It is also apparent that Sarah was able to withstand 28 severe events including trauma events before finally experiencing depression. So, this could indicate resilience to depression over a relatively long period of time. We also need to compare this careful detailing and unfolding of Sarah's scenario as helpful for understanding her situation for clinical work or targeted intervention by services. There may well have been opportunity for her to seek further help – whether legal, financial or psychotherapeutic which may have averted her depression. Clearly seeing her simply as a victim is much too simplistic; in this sense, she did survive for much of this lengthy episode and was very active in dealing with it. Presenting her solely as a victim of domestic violence may underplay both her active and persistent coping and the deviousness of her partner.

The importance of life history

Having a history of trauma sensitises individuals to developing PTSD (Brewin et al., 2000) and individuals suffering from PTSD are vulnerable to increased symptoms after subsequently experiencing a new trauma (Fossion et al., 2015; Hantman & Solomon, 2007). There are dose effects between trauma and the development of PTSD (Johnson & Thompson, 2008; Mollica, McInnes, Pool, & Tor, 1998); thus, the greater multiplicity of trauma experiences the higher the likelihood of PTSD resulting. This is important to consider given that trauma-tised patients have generally experienced several potentially traumatic events (Carey, Stein, Zungu-Dirwayi, & Seedat, 2003).

There is research literature surrounding the delayed effect on symptoms of some types of trauma (Schock et al., 2016). This occurs in some of the veteran literature (Horesh et al., 2011) where full PTSD may occur some years after combat experience when solders return to everyday life. They may however engage in substance abuse or have other types of symptoms in between. One example from the LEDS London Coping sample (see study 5, Appendix 1) was the story of a woman Mary whose trauma involved the death of her ten-year-old son who was playing on a building site and died three years before she was interviewed for our study. Mary had suffered from anxiety disorder as a result but did not get depressed despite her general distress and feelings of both guilt and blame. The trauma event had negative effects on her mar-riage, her other child's problematic behaviours and Mary's poor relationships with close family and friends. Then, in the course of the follow-up to our study, the school her son had attended held a memorial service for him, with her permission, which she attended. This event itself was not considered a severe life event, since it dealt with an anniversary which was being hon-oured and had no further practical ramifications. However, Mary became depressed soon after this event. It was as though this event had reawakened or resonated with the earlier trauma event and perhaps finally let her acknowl-edge and respond to her loss.

Links to prior trauma experience are further exemplified by child-hood trauma, which has the additional element of hindering psychologi-cal development in children and can exert long-lasting effects. This will be examined further in Chapter 4. Thus, a full exploration of both the na-ture of trauma experience and the inter-relationships with earlier trauma experiences is likely to be critical to understanding their effects. Those who only explore one or two exposures may miss the deleterious effects of co-occurring traumatic experience and underestimate the socio-environmental contribution. When these are ignored, researchers and clinicians may be-lieve that the presence of one type of adversity has the same effect in all cases (Dong et al., 2004). Therefore, understanding how an event sits within an in-dividual's life history, including the multiplicity and chronicity of any given traumatic event, may be of great importance in understanding trauma and may differentiate between individuals currently included as having trauma exposure.

Clinical implications

Understanding the full extent of trauma exposure can help clinicians when diagnosing and intervening with PTSD. The additional detail may point to aspects of cognitive-emotional response around Security, Identity and Attachment. The 'dose' of stress can be better understood when the multiples of trauma events are known, and when the aspects of loss, danger, humiliation and entrapment are understood. These individuals need to feel safe in the therapeutic situation; having had their fundamental life safety threatened, they need to know that they can trust the therapist to be able to open up to discuss painful experiences in their presence. However, there is acknowledgement that trauma responses do require a broader approach than 'talking cures', with effective interventions including those which have a physical basis (including exercise and meditation). We outline here two such approaches. The Comprehensive Resource model of trauma experience and Eye Movement Desensitisation Response (EMDR) which have had success with trauma responses.

Comprehensive resource model (CRM) and trauma experience

The CRM is a holistic therapeutic approach to help clients re-process and release the effects of traumatic events which they have experienced with a biological focus (Cohen & Mannarino, 2008). While using CRM techniques, a therapist helps their client learn a variety of techniques to build a neurological scaffolding of resources in the mid-brain, limbic system and neocortex. Issues described as the 'parts' inside us, which hold the trauma, are invited into a 'grid' which incorporates a wide range of tailored breathing skills, somatic embodiment skills, attachment neurobiology and spiritual resourcing to achieve its aims. This containment framework allows the client to feel sufficiently safe to retain a high level of consciousness during the reprocessing of their trauma and so avoid being re-traumatised or to dissociate, as can happen without a safety system such as this in place. Evaluation of this technique includes several randomised controlled trials, showing effectiveness in ongoing studies for children experiencing sexual abuse, domestic violence, traumatic grief, terrorism, disasters and multiple traumas (Cohen & Mannarino, 2008). The physical basis of the therapy and important safety awareness make this specific to traumatisation.

Eye movement desensitisation and reprocessing (EMDR)

EMDR is a psychotherapy treatment that was originally designed to alleviate the distress associated with traumatic memories (Shapiro, 2017). Shapiro's Adaptive Information Processing model posits that EMDR therapy facilitates the accessing and processing of traumatic memories and other adverse life experience to bring these to an adaptive resolution (Shapiro & Maxfield, 2002). It is argued that after successful treatment with EMDR therapy, affective distress is relieved, negative beliefs are reformulated and physiological arousal is reduced. During EMDR therapy, the client attends to emotionally disturbing material in brief sequential doses while simultaneously focusing on an external stimulus. Therapist-directed lateral eye movements are the most commonly used external stimulus (e.g. the client follows the therapists' slow-moving finger in front of their eyes), but a variety of other stimuli including hand-tapping and audio stimulation are often used (Shapiro, 1991). The working hypothesis is that EMDR therapy facilitates the accessing of the traumatic memory network often not accessible in 'talking cures' so that information processing is enhanced, with new associations forged between the traumatic memory and more adaptive memories or information. These new associations are thought to result in completed information processing, new learning, elimination of emotional distress and development of cognitive insights. EMDR therapy uses a three pronged protocol: (1) the past events that have laid the groundwork for dysfunction are processed, forging new associative links with adaptive information; (2) the current circumstances that elicit distress are targeted and internal and external triggers are desensitised; and (3) imagined templates of future events are incorporated to assist the client in acquiring the skills needed for adaptive functioning.[1]

A study evaluating the relative efficacy of EMDR compared to a no-treatment waitlist control (WAIT) in the treatment of PTSD in adult female rape victims (Rothbaum, 1997). Improvement in PTSD depression, dissociation, and state anxiety was significantly greater in the EMDR than the WAIT group (Rothbaum, 1997). Other studies have also shown positive impacts (Lee, Gavriel, Drummond, Richards, & Greenwald, 2002).

Clinical challenges and discussion

Challenges in treating individuals with PTSD involve their frequent inability to speak of their trauma. This is thought to be related to a physiological impact in those traumatised with decreased activity in the Broca's area in the left frontal lobe of the cortex. This is the speech centre of the brain, often also adversely affected in stroke victims, where blood supply to the area is cut off. Without this part of the brain functioning, the individual cannot put their thoughts and feelings into words. Scans of PTSD patients show that the Broca's area is deactivated whenever a flashback is triggered rending the individual temporarily in the state of a stroke victim (Cozolino, 2005; van der Kolk, 2001). This together with the fact that some childhood trauma experience is pre-verbal may account for why many individuals cannot speak about their trauma even years later. Even when people do manage to narrate what happened to them, these accounts are rarely coherent and don't always convey the inner 'truth' despite the fact that sensations, sounds and images may be stored in memory. This brings to mind the quote: 'for most of it I have no words' from a CBS correspondent on viewing the horror of concentration camps at the end of the Second World War (van der Kolk, 2015, p. 43).

The 'frozen' response where individuals are unable to access the memory, thoughts and feelings around the trauma events they have experienced can inhibit the clinical healing process. This involves a form of denial where the body may register the threat, but the conscious mind does not register it. Yet, simultaneously, the body's alarm system continues, and the stress hormones keep sending signals to the muscles for 'flight or fight'. Medications, drugs or alcohol can be used to quell these unpleasant sensations, but the more enduring intervention is to 'unlock' these experiences making them accessible to the client.

The clinician has two particular challenges: getting individuals to desensitise to the past, but also to help them live fully and securely in the present. They also need to contend with the fact that the past trauma cannot in itself be 'undone'. What needs to be countered is the impacts of fear of losing control, of being on the constant alert for danger or rejection, for the self-loathing or blocks to engaging fully (van der Kolk, 2015). Recovery requires what is termed 'gaining ownership of the self – mind and body' (op cit, p. 203), thus to become calm and focused, to maintain that calm (even through an intrusive flashback), to be fully alive in the present and engaged with others and not keeping secrets. This may require revisiting the trauma and confronting it without being overwhelmed by sensations and memories of the past.

In conclusion, we believe that trauma events reflect the extreme on a life event spectrum of magnitude and can be tied to context in the same way in exploring their damaging nature. Characteristics such as loss, danger, humiliation and entrapment can potentially be applied to trauma event categorisations to further specify their key characteristics. These attributes may be crucial in refining our understanding of not only why some events are considered traumatic but also their specific impacts. For instance, it may help to understand the likely repercussions of a traumatic loss on symptomatology when compared to traumatic danger with humiliation that may occur from partner violence.

In addition, we have argued the critical importance of current and longer-term context, especially as negative experiences including traumatic events tend to cluster within individuals and their effects can have multiple and cumulative impacts. Critically, traumatic experiences are rarely isolated events, and the unique impact of any given trauma may be difficult to ascertain. We believe that a dimensional approach to characteristics of trauma taken from life events research could have potential for greater clarification of trauma event attributes and severity. This could have direct implications for more person-focused treatment of trauma, whereby individual context is taken into account.

Note

1 https://www.emdr.com/what-is-emdr/

4 Life events and vulnerability

Whilst most of us suffer adversity whether in the form of severe life events, or trauma events, relatively few us of suffer emotional disorder. Therefore, not all severe events lead to disorder. There are factors which make some of us more susceptible than others. Such susceptibility (or vulnerability) is very individual, made up of our ways of thinking and feeling, based on our memories of early life and the expectations derived as well as our neurobiology. It dictates how we appraise the events that occur, how we cope with them, who we talk to about them and how we judge their likely impact on our lives going forward. For some, engrained negative appraisal of experience leads to long-term pessimistic, hopeless and self-berating or blaming responses to life's hardships. Where mistrust is embedded, it creates unwillingness to seek help and solace at time of need. This chapter will seek to outline various aspects of vulnerability to emotional disorder.

Vulnerability spans the life course. *Proximal* vulnerability factors are those recent and ongoing in adults present when experiencing the severe life events that may bring about clinical disorder. It is linked through mediating or linking factors to early life experience which includes childhood trauma and maltreatment experience. These latter are termed *distal* vulnerability factors. The two are related, but can appear in different forms (e.g. distal maybe experiences of childhood neglect or abuse or social deprivation, proximal maybe insecure attachment style or cognitive helplessness or low self-esteem). Both types of vulnerability have been investigated through multi-disciplinary approaches – psychological (cognitive-affective and interpersonal), sociological (prior adverse environments) and biological (genetic and neurobiological factors). The overview presented here can only skim over a complex and wide-ranging area but will hopefully elucidate the conditions under which some individuals develop lifelong susceptibility to the effects of stressful life events to experience emotional disorder. First is a description of proximal vulnerability.

Proximal vulnerability

This section will focus on the psychological impacts which affect thinking and emotion and which can create negative biases that impede adult coping with stressors. This will encompass attachment models with a focus on close support, and the cognitive distortions that can come about through childhood maltreatment and early life adversity, particularly low self-esteem. Early findings from the Brown and Harris team showed lack of close support as a key adult vulnerability factor. A cross-sectional study in Camberwell (study 1, Appendix 1) identified lack of intimacy, defined as having no close confiding with partner or any close other seen regularly, as a key factor raising the likelihood of depression once a severe life event was encountered (Brown & Harris, 1978). This was interpreted as likely to relate to negative feelings about the self, as well as interpersonal relating problems, and both factors were later tested as vulnerability factors for depression. Taking inspiration from the Beck model of depression with its negative cognitive biases, the Bedford Square team focused on low self-esteem as an underlying vulnerability factor. The Self-Esteem and Social Support (SESS) interview was designed specifically to look at vulnerability through a number of subjective scales about the self and others focused more externally reflecting identity and security as well as close confiding relationships (O'Connor & Brown, 1984). This was first tested in a prospective investigation of Islington working-class mothers (study 3, Appendix 1) (Brown, Andrews, Bifulco, & Veiel, 1990). This led to exploration of self-esteem as a construct and to a number of key findings about self-esteem and its association with close supportive relationships and depression.

Having initially measured a large number of scales about the self, a factor analysis of ten scales reflecting aspects of self-worth (self-acceptance, self-attributes and evaluation of personal role performance, both positive and negative aspects) as well as those focused more widely (scales of security, meaningfulness, control and satisfaction of life) indicated these grouped into three factors – negative self-evaluation, positive self-evaluation and the satisfaction/meaning scales. An index was derived of negative evaluation of self (NES) which included a high (marked or moderate) rating of negative self-attributes (such as feeling stupid or unattractive or negative role-attributes (report of being a bad mother or incompetent worker) and low (some or little/no) self-acceptance (feeling of being unworthy). The three scales were combined and dichotomised as an index (NES) which was rated as 'present' if any one of those negatively rated dimensions was rated highly.

Example of NES

This woman reported 'marked' negative self-evaluation (comments from the full interview listed together):

> 'When I get dressed up and have my hair styled I sometimes feel a bit attractive but that's not very often.'
> 'I am efficient some of the time in the flat but I often muddle through'. .....
> 'I am a bit of a loner, I'm described by others as that clean woman with the drinking problem, but I'm not always that clean...'
> 'I'm not very educated; I can't answer questions like that – I'm not intelligent. I was never bright' (She repeated this in response to a number of

questions). She explains that she needed remedial teaching when at school but never got it. 'I'm not able to do even simple jobs. I haven't got the intelligence, I'm stupid. I washed up in a restaurant (as a part-time job) with two different sized plates - no matter how often I was told, I kept mixing them up. So I just gave up with work. I was always very slow in my actions. I'm too old to care now" [She is in fact aged 42, but perceives herself as much older].

'I'm moody. I think I'm sympathetic, but I've turned a bit hard. If my father died, I wouldn't go to his funeral. I wouldn't care'. She finds it hard to say what she thinks. 'I'm not direct. I'm not direct with my husband. I'm easy-going. I let him get away with a lot.'

The first analysis to explore correlates of NES used a continuous NES score, summing the full four-point ratings on each of the three negative scales (Brown, Bifulco, Veiel, Andrews, 1990). Predictors were then examined in relation to a range of other scales involving relationships and roles. Those significantly predictive of NES included negative interaction with close others (arguments or rows with child or partner or with other close relationships), social isolation (lacking social contacts or close others) and security decreasing character of housework (seeing it as a drudge and detrimental to self). Other scales that included lack of resources (those financial, social, employment and close ties outside the household) did not contribute to predicting NES. The outcome of this exploratory work was the construction of two indices – one reflecting negative self and the other negative close relationships.

The NES index was examined prospectively to new onset of depression (Brown, Bifulco, & Andrews, 1990a), together with the second index of Negative Elements in Close Relationships (NECR) which was made up of interpersonal scales including lack of close confiding support or negative interaction with partner or children. These together were tested prospectively in relation to new onsets of depression. Combination of the two indices NES and NECR resulted in more than fourfold (46% vs 10%) risk of major depression when severe events were encountered (Bifulco, Brown, Moran, Ball, & Campbell, 1998) and thus identified as proximal vulnerability factors (see Figure 4.1).

One of the most pertinent findings from these studies is the statistical *interaction* between vulnerability and severe life event (the model shows a Relative Risk of 45.8) in increasing the likelihood of new onset. Furthermore, other important linkages are indicated – for example, severe event alone is 13 times more likely to bring about onset of depression, and vulnerability alone is 10 times more likely. A further prospective study (Coping study 5, Appendix 1) which selected only women with these vulnerability factors who were free from depression at first contact showed more than 75% of them experienced a severe life event in the follow-up year. Moreover, many of these events had the negative characteristics and dimensions discussed in the last chapter, suggesting a higher link between vulnerability and experiencing severe life events (Bifulco et al., 1998). In this later study, 48% of women with a severe event developed a new onset of clinical depression (op cit).

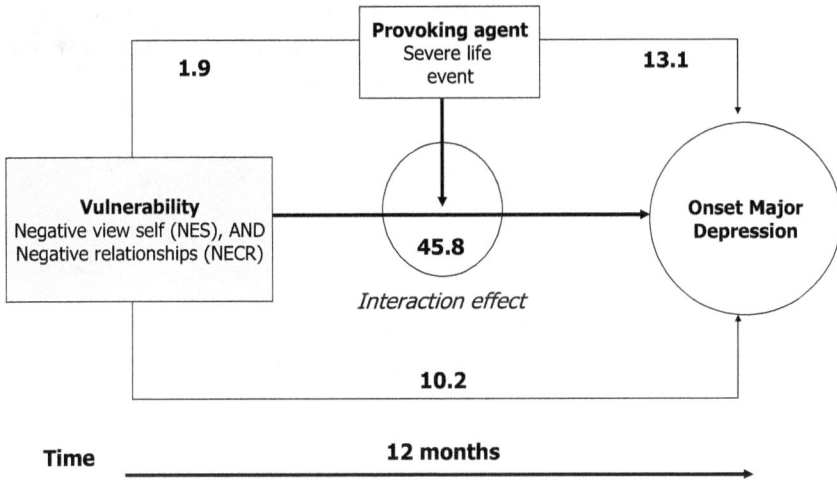

Figure 4.1 Model of vulnerability provoking agent and onset of depression. (Relative risks shown).

In order to understand why both NECR and negative self-evaluation provided the best index of proximal vulnerability, an overarching attachment framework was invoked. This utilised the concept of insecure attachment style as key to a vulnerability profile, related to patterns of low support through isolation or conflict in relationships as well as low self-esteem (Bifulco, Moran, Ball, & Bernazzani, 2002). Following the theoretical approaches of John Bowlby and Mary Ainsworth, attachment frameworks bring together a range of social experience to influence lifetime risk of disorder through poor ability to relate to close others which leads to an absence of social support in time of need (Cassidy & Shaver, 1999). The attachment framework has now been adopted internationally both in research and service development, and further supported by studies from around the world. It has shown that early childhood experiences of negative parenting lead to changes in the individual's habitual thinking and feeling (cognitive-affective templates) which endure and then determine responses to making and maintaining close relationships in adult life. Whereas secure style is adaptive and normative, those insecure styles denoting anxious or avoidant characteristics lead to different types of difficulty in relating to others. Such styles are known to be associated with a range of psychological disorders (Bartholomew & Horowitz, 1991; Belsky & Nezworski, 1987; Berry, Barrowclough, & Wearden, 2007) and have also been investigated in Canada and the USA in relation to physical illness such as diabetes (Ciechanowski, Katon, Russo, & Dwight-Johnson, 2002) and barriers to service-use (Maunder, 2009).

The Attachment Style Interview (ASI) was developed by the Bedford Square team to find a practical way of measuring such styles based solely on current attitudes and behaviours in relationships. This moved away from the more psychodynamic way of measuring attachment style through coherence in report-ing of childhood memories (Main & Cassidy, 1988). The ASI proved to be a highly reliable and transparent method of categorising attachment based on the quality of close supportive relationships. This included responses to questions about close confiding, emotional support and quality of interaction with partner and two or three very close others as well as attitudes around mistrust, fear of rejection or separation, self-reliance and anger (Bifulco & Thomas, 2012). See Figure 4.2 for the overall style profiles.

Clearly Secure (lack of negative attitudes, good relationships)

This is the most stable and flexible style with a lack of negative attitudes denoting either anxious or avoidant attachment. There is comfort with closeness and appropriate levels of autonomy. There will always be 'good' ('marked or moderate') ability to make and maintain relationships and evidence of good support.

Anxious attachment styles

Enmeshed: (High fear of separation)

This is a dependent attachment style as exhibited by high Desire for Company, and low Self-reliance and high Fear of Separation. These individuals tend to have fairly superficial relationships and despite a high number of social contacts may have few which are objectively close. Anger is sometimes present, denoting the Ambivalence often associated with this style.

Fearful: (High fear of rejection)This attachment style has fears of being rejected or let down which is generalised to others. This may relate to actual experiences of having been let down which have generalized to fear of future interactions. There is often a desire to get close to others, together with fear of doing so which can lead to loneliness. Fearful style will always have '1: Marked' or '2: Moderate' on Fear of Rejection, and is the only style that rates high on this scale. Anger is absent.

Avoidant attachment styles

Angry-Dismissive (High mistrust and Anger)

This style is characterised by high Mistrust, high Self-reliance and low Desire for Company. Its key characteristic is high Anger. Individuals with this style usually need a high level of control over their lives, are extremely self-reliant and typically are in conflict with those around them. This is often reflected in individual interactions with close others and family as well as in feelings of anger and resentment about the past.

Withdrawn: (High self-reliance)

This is a detached style characterised by high Self-reliance, high Constraints on Closeness and low Desire for Company. This is often expressed as desire for privacy and clear boundaries with

---

Figure 4.2 Summary of ASI attachment styles. (Bifulco & Thomas, 2012, pp. 37–38).

regard to others. However, there is neither fear nor anger expressed. It can appear as very practical, rational and non-emotional style.

Anxious and Avoidant style

Disorganised Insecure: This dual attachment classification is only considered for those rated 'markedly' or 'moderately' insecure; it has no secure counterpart. It reflects those individuals who are unable to relate to others and for whom no single clear style can be determined from the subscales rated. Both 'primary' and 'subsidiary' attachment styles are rated with precedence given to the more pervasive style which affects wider relationships. An example of dual rating is when a high degree of both anger and fear in relationships fulfil both Angry-dismissive and either Fearful or Enmeshed types. Enmeshed and Fearful can also be included and unusually Enmeshed and Withdrawn. The autonomy scales (self-reliance and desire for company) may be rated as 'contradictory' to show the pull in both anxious and avoidant directions.

Figure 4.2 Continued.

Insecure attachment style categories were rated on a continuum of 'marked', 'moderate' or 'some' level of the style selected according to the cognitive-affective profile. This proved instructive since only the 'marked' or 'moderate' levels of style related to depression. 'Mild' levels of insecure anxious as well as the specific Withdrawn style had no higher rates of depression than those secure (Bifulco et al., 2002). When prevalence was examined (study 5 Coping and 6 Sisters combined, Appendix 1), it could be seen that around 24% of comparison women studied had a highly insecure style and 47% with other vulnerability (op cit).

Insecure attachment style was shown in adult women to relate both to childhood neglect and abuse and to adult major depression (Bifulco, Moran, Ball, & Lillie, 2002). Insecure attachment style was also shown in a prospective study to mediate between the two (Bifulco et al., 2006) for new onsets of depression and anxiety disorder. The styles most clearly mediating were Fearful style and Angry-dismissive style. Hence, women experiencing childhood neglect and abuse, who also had the adult vulnerability of either Fearful or Angry-dismissive style, were more likely to experience onsets of depression and anxiety disorder than women with other styles. Withdrawn style was unrelated to either childhood experience or depression, and Enmeshed style had some inconsistency in results. This is because Enmeshed style, less common in the London sample, seemed also less likely to emerge from childhood neglect or abuse, but rather from childhood parental loss and antipathy (cold, critical parenting) (Bifulco & Thomas, 2012). Further analysis of attachment style in adulthood showed insecure styles significantly related to low self-esteem or NES (Bifulco et al, 2002) as well as NECR – lack of close support and conflictful relationships. They also related to domestic violence (Bifulco, Damiani, Jacobs, & Spence, 2019; Bifulco et al., 2002). Those with insecure attachment styles also experienced more severe life events not only in relationships but also in finance and housing, and they were also shown to cope more poorly with such stressors (Bifulco & Thomas, 2012).

Insecure attachment style is thus an effective marker of adult vulnerability and shown to relate to adverse circumstances as well as disorder. This is illustrated below.

Sarah's vulnerable profile

In the last chapter, Sarah's situation was described and her trauma experience resulting from violence from her husband Steve, the actions she took to expel him from the household and her attempts to pay back his debts. It also outlines how, at certain points, she allowed him back into her flat and later went on holiday with him even though this led to more violence. Here, we look at her proximal vulnerability which may have led to her initial involvement with him and contributed to her perseverance in trying to mend the relationship despite the risks of harm.

Sarah was identified for study (Coping project, study 5, Appendix 1) with vulnerable characteristics when selected but free then from depression. She reported by questionnaire her negative interaction with her husband and children and her lack of close confidants (NECR present). This was confirmed at interview. However, she did not have NES – in fact, she had a positive view of herself and her capabilities. She said:

> I am confident. I can be quite demanding, but only demanding in what's right for the family. I do nag a bit, but find I am justified. I'm very truthful – I'm always 100%. I'd describe myself as fairly easy going, helpful, caring person. I wish I could be stronger at times – I'm a soft touch. I feel I've got to be strong the whole time (as a mother). I would never put myself down.

Much of her NECR focused on her partner relationship. When first seen, she described her relationship with her partner as difficult. When asked if she talked to him about problems, she elaborated:

> 'The problems are usually involving him!' *(Talk to him?)* 'Oh yes, but you see he's got me on this pedestal that nothing ever goes wrong for me – and that there's always something wrong with him. If I say I'm ill, I don't get much back.' *(Confide in him?)* 'Yeah, but if it gets too hot for him and he knows I'm getting near the bone, that I'm right, then – like last night – I was trying to talk to him and he just stormed off to bed."Oh I'm not taking any more of this" he said. Because he doesn't want bad things said to him.' When she tried telling him about her problems at work he comments: "oh I'm sick of hearing this" and just leaves.

It transpired later in the interview that her partner did keep things from her like his drink-driving court case:

'He makes me feel like I'm a real dragon or something, that he doesn't want to tell me'. (*Make you feel bad about yourself?*) 'Yes definitely – he's made me feel like I don't know whether I'm coming or going. You know, one minute I think I'm better off without him, and then he can just change, like he took us away to Folkestone for the bank holiday. You get a bit of confidence in him and you think 'oh he's doing alright by us' and then he lets you down again and again. And I feel it's not fair to do that to the children. You can't do it, I don't like that.'

She also had negative interactions with her partner, and she described him as very jealous as he accused her of having affairs:

'Sometimes he's made me feel as if it's me and I start thinking, is it me? Have I gone mad? I think what he does, it's like somebody trying to manipulate you, and he tries to make you feel as though it's partly your fault. And then I think well maybe it is my fault, but then I think about things and I think, no, it's not my fault! Funnily enough, I had a chat with him on Monday night and he shouted 'what is going wrong with us?' I said, 'Steve, *you* are what is going wrong with us at the moment. I've always been the same person.' He tries to make you think it's you, you see. He doesn't want to take the responsibility for anything. I said don't try and shift the blame this time, you've done it for years. I know it's not my fault. I've been very positive about that.

I had a row with him last night funnily enough. I slept here [sofa] and he slept in the bedroom. I just didn't want to be in the same bed. It's because of the way he's been [with drink and drugs] and he won't talk about things. It was basically because we had a row [Sarah didn't want sex] and he puts a lot of importance on sex. I fight with him about that. But I mean, I enjoy it as much as him. He sulks if he doesn't get sex, and I think, for god's sake! And as I said, funnily enough I said to him 'you seem to put so much importance on that. Can't you accept me and sometimes I might not want sex?' Then he actually threatened me, he said, 'well if this carries on for much longer I'll go elsewhere.' Well, I said, 'you can go elsewhere and that'll be the end of my problems!' [laughs].

Sarah had only one support figure – a close confidant seen every couple of months. She also named a close friend in Scotland but she was not a confidant and not seen regularly. Sarah thus has little emotional support close to hand. Her attachment style proved at interview to be 'moderately' Angry-dismissive. This was signalled by her lack of close support and her argumentative relationship with her partner and anger towards her children. She also reported a high level of mistrust of others, being overly self-reliant and angry at those around her.

It is notable she described herself, and advocated being 'strong' which is a common theme among individuals with this style.

When asked about mistrust, she explained her suspiciousness and why she avoided certain friends at the moment:

> A lot of it is, they tend to tell me things, like, perhaps about Steve, you know, 'Oh, he was doing this or he was doing that,' knowing that it's going to wind me up or something, and I do get wound up very easily. But I don't like being told lies, I like the truth, I've been brought up that way and I just can't change. I just don't like people telling lies. (*About her husband's infidelity*) I'm not a suspicious person, but once someone's done something like that I'm very mistrusting, but anybody would be, I suppose. But I shut it out of my mind, but then when he came in with a love-bite on his neck, flaunting it sort of thing. I really.... that was a terrible time.

When asked about having 'constraints on closeness', in relation to confiding and help-seeking, she commented:

> I always seem to attract these sort of people (who take but don't give). I don't know why it is. But they always have hang-ups, problems, and I feel sorry for them. But I don't realise how bad the problems are until I get involved. I've hidden a lot from Steve and other people, I suppose because not many people, like at my work, know that he's ever hit me. It's not the sort of thing I would go round telling people anyway. I haven't told anyone about how bad he can be. I would rather hold things back.

She described herself as always relying on herself not others. She feels she has had to struggle with her own problems and with everyone else's and usually without any help. She also shows anger in terms of resentment to friends:

> (Her close friend) 'I tended to do a lot for her, she had me running around all over the place with her. I thought to myself, this is ridiculous, you know, she and her family are always coming down to me for meals and there was never any returning. I thought, she's just using me, you know. I got to the stage where I thought, hang on here, I'm the one with three children and need support. And I just thought, no, because people do take advantage, because I am very good-natured.' (*Is it only her?*) 'Oh no, it's a few people who have taken advantage.'

As well as having arguments with her husband and resentments towards friends, she also loses her patience with her children:

> 'They tend to...like I say, if I want to go to the toilet or something they won't leave me alone. They have got to have me there. It is like everyone depends

on me the whole time, and I'm not feeling sorry for myself but, for support, I do like a bit of attention, everybody does, and a bit of acknowledgement rather than 'can I have this mum, can I have that mum, mum,' that sort of thing does annoy me'. (*Do you lose temper with them?*) 'Yes, and then if I've got to keep telling them to do things, that annoys me. Oh that happens quite a lot, like telling them to do things, that annoys me– you are shouting in the end.'

Sarah's vulnerability is thus focused more on how she manages her relationships rather than on her feelings of self-worth. In fact, she expects a lot of herself – to be self-reliant, strong and manage without help from other people. However, living with an abusive husband has eroded some of her self-belief and has led her to mistrust all he tells her. The stigma associated with an abusive relationship also makes her cautious about telling other people about her problems with her husband. She therefore bottles it up and tries to manage alone with what are fairly effective practical coping strategies.

Despite an array of life events, Sarah still seems to have hope that the relationship with her husband will come right. With the severe life events listed in the last chapter, it can be seen that she eventually becomes depressed only after an attempted reconciliation when they go on holiday together. However, this too led to violence. Eventually, after 18 months of marital and financial difficulty resulting from her husband's behaviour, she feels that she can no longer hold herself together.

We can track Sarah's psychosocial vulnerabilities back to her early life experiences which will be outlined later in this chapter. It becomes clear from examining the quotes from the interview above that some key features of these proximal vulnerabilities include her belief in her own strength to deal with any situation and her mistrust that others can help. This has been effective in her life for large tranches of time, but in her current very stressful situation, it no longer enables her to cope. It should of course be added that her husband's antisocial behaviour and efforts to undermine her are also feeding into her coping responses.

To anticipate the discussion later in this chapter, we can also identify some of the important events in her childhood experience that added to her adult vulnerability. Her upbringing in Scotland involved neglect from her parents. They were unconcerned about her wellbeing, did not let her discuss problems and took little interest in her schoolwork or friendships. They gave her little attention or time. It was a household which maintained high discipline and her parents were not affectionate. She did, however, get some care and affection from her paternal grandmother whom she visited often.

However, an early trauma experience involved sexual abuse from her paternal grandfather when she visited her grandmother. This happened when she was aged nine. He would ask her to come into his bed and kiss him and would offer her money. He also used to tell her about his previous sexual encounters. Sarah felt upset on behalf of her grandmother. The situation worsened from when she was 13 and continued for two years. She recalls:

> At 13, I remember he took out his thing (penis) one night and I was just petrified, and I ran away but I couldn't tell my grandmother because it would upset her too much. He would try to get me to touch him, but I wouldn't let him – I knew it was wrong. He exposed himself about five times from when I was 13. It was more a cry for help that I told my mum. Then when my dad confronted him, and he denied it, I was accused of being a liar which was awful. After that my grandfather just said I was "asking for it" that I was the one doing all the leading....

She left home early at age 16 to come to London with a friend and managed to find work and accommodation. She met Steve after 18 months and they moved in together when she was aged 19. She described the relationship as close at first – but he became involved in criminal activity, and they were separated when he went to prison for armed robbery. She described an episode of depression around this time. She returned to Scotland, and when Steve was released from prison, they lived together again in London and Sarah got pregnant. They then married. When she was pregnant with her second child (which was unplanned), Steve announced that he wanted to leave her and live abroad. He became violent at this point which was the only episode of violence prior to the recent one. He later spent more time in prison. When he came out of prison, they continue to live together and have a third child.

Sarah's history shows how early life trauma and neglect can be linked to her angry-dismissive attachment style with its elements of mistrust and self-reliance. This vulnerability is also added to by adult adversity which includes partnership with an unreliable and criminal and violent husband, and periods of lone parenthood while he is in prison. She meets him having gone to live in a distant city aged only 16, without any family support, and despite positive coping in relation to finding work and somewhere to live, she gets involved with a dangerous man. What stands out in the account is the extent to which she persists in the relationship with him despite his prison sentences and the periods of separation. This may be because she has a determination to be strong and has perhaps unrealistic expectations of her own coping and ability to change him. It may also indicate some gullibility in her judgements about others. There may also have been instances of coercive control from her partner which may have reduced her ability to escape the relationship.

Biological sources of proximal vulnerability

The next section will now look at another aspect of proximal vulnerability – that emanating from biological sources. Two aspects will be highlighted – first the direct relationship of genes governing serotonin production, and the relationship to depression when interacting with severe life events. This is considered a gene ×

environment (G × E) relationship. The second aspect concerns biological correlates of insecure attachment style including cortisol (stress hormone).

Serotonin and severe life events

The field of behavioural genomics has examined target genes associated with vulnerability to psychological disorder. Thus, it is argued, underlying genetic factors may influence a person's biological response to different environmental factors – specifically make them more sensitised to the experience of certain severe life events. Serotonin production in particular has been highlighted as a factor related to mood and emotion. Researchers believe that an imbalance in serotonin levels may influence mood in a way that leads to depression (Cowen, 2002). Possible problems include low brain cell production of serotonin, a lack of receptor sites able to receive the serotonin that is made, inability of serotonin to reach the receptor sites or a shortage in tryptophan, the chemical from which serotonin is made. If any of these biochemical glitches occur, researchers believe that it can lead to both depression and anxiety (Cowen & Browning, 2015).

The gene which has been a focus of research, and one associated with depression, is the serotonin transporter gene SLC6A4 and its associated polymorphism (Bleys, Luyten, Soenens, & Claes, 2018). Serotonin is a neurotransmitter affecting a number of physiological processes as well as cognitive brain functions including mood and emotions. Thus, low serotonin levels have been linked with depressed mood which has led in turn to treatments involving selective serotonin reuptake inhibitors (SSRIs) commonly prescribed as antidepressants. In particular, the 5-HTTLPR polymorphism in the promoter region of the serotonin transporter gene has been a focus for research on its links to depression. 'Genetic polymorphism' means that different people might have slight variations in their DNA at a specific location in the genome which could affect how well the protein and the gene are effective. In the case of 5-HTTLPR, there is both a short (s) and a long allele (l) – the former being more common in those with depression. It is therefore hypothesised that those individuals with the short 's' allele may be more likely to develop depression when experiencing severe life events.

Various studies have been conducted to support this hypothesis although findings have been varied (Fisher et al., 2012; Risch et al., 2009; Uher & McGuffin, 2008, 2010). Risch and colleagues included 14 studies in their meta-analysis of G × E and only included those that assessed severe life events in interaction with 5HTTLPR (Risch et al., 2009). They found that the number of severe life events was associated with depression but found no evidence for the association either between depression itself and the serotonin transporter gene or for the interaction between life events, 5-HTTLPR and depression, thus failing to support the hypothesis of moderation and G × E. This was confirmed by a collaborative meta-analysis which conducted standardised analyses on date from 31 studies (Culverhouse et al., 2018). One explanation for inconsistency in findings is provided by Brown and colleagues who argue that the chronicity of the depression is critical – thus showing impacts of 5-HTTLPR on episodes which took a chronic course (of 12 months duration or longer) rather than those acute (Brown et al., 2013). (See further discussion below under childhood vulnerability.)

However, other explanations of inconsistent findings for this genetic polymorphism implicate the type of measurement used for life events. Thus, it is reported that the expected interaction was found more often with studies using more intensive measures such as the LEDS (Uher & McGuffin, 2010). The different strategies used in meta-analysis for study inclusion and meta-analytic statistical techniques have also been identified as potentially changing overall conclusions (Taylor & Munafò, 2016). This was evidenced by reworking of a more inclusive meta-analysis by Karg and colleagues (Karg, Burmeister, Shedden, & Sen, 2011). Whereas the latter did find a significant interaction using a different technique, this was not then replicated (Taylor & Munafò, 2016). This indicates that scrutiny of different methodologies and measures may help to shed light on ways in which these genetic, physiological and psychological processes do or do not interact. It also illustrates that the methodology and measures used are important in shedding light on the way in which these genetic, physiological and psychological processes interact.

Another focus of research explored the influence of a common single-nucleotide polymorphism (Val66Met), so named because it is a brain-derived neurotrophic factor (BDNF) gene, a methionine (Met) substitution for valine (Val) at codon 66 (Val66Met). This is associated with alterations in brain anatomy and memory, hypothesised to relate to clinical disorder (Anastasia et al., 2013). Brown led a team investigating the nature in which the functional Val66Met polymorphism of BDNF interacts with recent severe life events to produce onsets of new depressive episodes. Utilising the LEDS to identify severe life events, the study brought together women from a range of prior studies (see study 10, Appendix 1) to obtain valid BDNF genotypes (Brown et al., 2013). Results showed that Met alleles of BDNF moderated the relationship between recent life events and adult onsets of depression in a significant gene–environment interaction, thus supporting the hypothesis.

Thus, proximal vulnerability has been identified as involving cognitive (self-esteem), interpersonal (attachment style) and genetic (serotonin gene-related) factors. The following discussion will be around distal vulnerability emanating from childhood experience.

Distal vulnerability

Most of the theoretical approaches to vulnerability chart its course from childhood adverse experience. These approaches focus on three possible pathways or strands of vulnerability (see Figure 4.4). First, studies which look at the 'dose' effects of varied adversity in childhood taking a sociological pathway from childhood adversity to adulthood involving perpetuated deprivation, social exclusion and adverse circumstances flowing from a disadvantaged start in life (Rutter, 1985a). This pathway is thought to generate severe life events and long-term problems with diminishing social and material resources for later coping and support, thus increasing stress with reduced resource.

The second psychological pathway involves the cognitive schemata implied in both Beck's negative cognitive triad and Bowlby's insecure attachment styles. Here, the 'latent schemata' are caused by childhood adversity. These are cognitive-affective processes which introduce negative biases into perception and can persist into adulthood. They reflect impeded psychological development and the cognitive (thinking) and affective (emotional) responses growing up, which can become enduring and activated at times of later stress. As previously discussed, such negative beliefs include that the world is dangerous, the future is hopeless, the self is unlovable and people are untrustworthy. This pathway is easily understood as a response in the face of gross deprivation and victimisation in childhood but which becomes maladaptive when ossified in later contexts (Bowlby, 1977).

Finally, the third, biological strand represents the neurobiological physical correlates of early life adversity which add to the weighting of vulnerability for the growing adult when encountering stressful conditions (McCrory, De Brito, & Viding, 2012) (see Figure 4.3). This includes genetic factors, impeded brain development, as well as cortisol dysregulation as a function of early life stress. Each of these strands will be examined in turn.

Childhood social adversity

Socio-environmental factors, leaning on Bronfenbrenner's socio-ecological model, include a range of experiences such as loss of parent, childhood poverty,

Psychosocial lifespan model of disorder

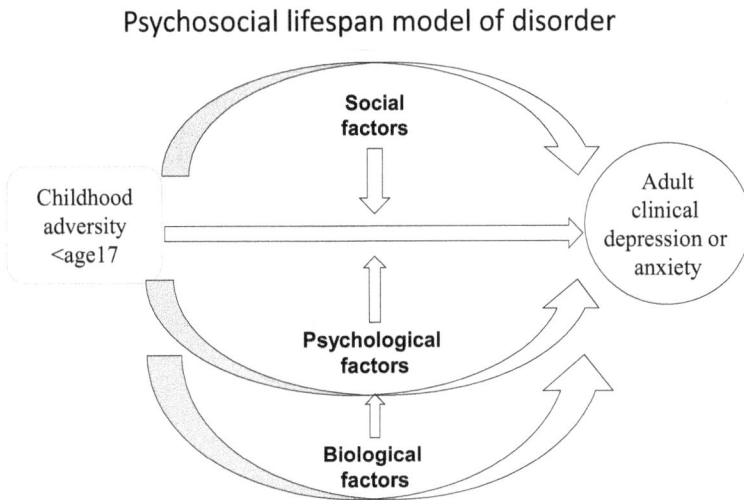

Figure 4.3 Psychosocial lifespan model of disorder.

parental illness and domestic violence, all of which have been associated with a range of poor health outcomes in the offspring – both physical (Leserman, Drossman, Li, Toomey et al., 1996) and psychological (Fergusson, Boden, & Horwood, 2008). Brown and Harris' early work showed that childhood experience, particularly around parental loss and problem care, is associated with a range of such adult risk factors including perpetuated lower socio-economic status, single parenthood and domestic violence, worse education and poorer employment record (Harris, Brown, & Bifulco, 1987). All of these speak to contemporary policy issues around child poverty and housing, family break-up, family conflict and its effect on children's development and wellbeing (Department of Work and Pensions, 2015). The issues of parental loss, financial hardship and parental illness will be outlined further.

Investigation of maternal loss in childhood has a long history and led, over 50 years ago, to the development of two different models – the earlier psychological one of attachment disruption (Bowlby, 1951) followed by a sociological one highlighting social deprivation (Rutter, 1972). In fact, both are supported, but indicate different pathways in mental health models. Brown and Harris' first model of depression in Camberwell, London found that individuals who lost a mother before age 11 had a much increased rate of depression as adults (Brown & Harris, 1978). This led to further investigation in North London samples, comparing individuals with different types of parental loss in childhood and lifetime depression. Whilst the association was confirmed with both depression and later disadvantage (Harris et al., 1987), the analysis also indicated that there was a mediating role of parental lack of care of the child (Bifulco, Brown, & Harris, 1987). Therefore, in the instance of death of mother, the psychoanalytic hypothesis of mourning and depression was unsupported with childhood mourning behaviours unrelated to adult depression (Bifulco, Harris, & Brown, 1992), whereas parental problem care and neglect that could arise after losing a mother had a much larger effect.

Childhood poverty has many long-term consequences for children, with lower childhood family income associated with lower earnings and poorer physical health (Duncan, Kalil, & Ziol-Guest, 2013). The Family Stress Model (Conger & Elder, 1994) posits that low family income leads to economic stress, adding to parental distress and conflict, both of which can then cause parenting problems. Thus, lower socio-economic status is associated with child maltreatment (Drake & Jonson-Reid, 2014). For example, economic factors, including unemployment and material hardship, significantly predict physical abuse (Conrad-Hiebner & Scanlon, 2015) with estimates, suggesting that they account for 27% of all child maltreatment (Doidge et al., 2017). An analysis by the Bedford Square team of the London Sisters sample (see study 6, Appendix 1), a community sample, half of whom were selected for childhood adversity, indicated significant associations between childhood poverty and later financial problems and depression (Spence, Nunn, & Bifulco, 2019). A more complex model demonstrated that physical abuse and shame mediated some of the relationship between childhood poverty and adult depression.

Children in families with parental emotional disorder experience more acute stressful events in childhood, particularly those of an interpersonal nature, than children with parents who have other problems such as medical illnesses (Barnes & Stein, 2000). These emotional health problems may be due to existing spousal difficulties or by prior conditions in the family such as poverty or conflict. These mental health difficulties in parents also relate to other family difficulties such as financial hardship and parental loss (Barnes et al., 2005). Psychiatric disorder in the parent can act as a magnet for familial stress, which in turn can perpetuate the conditions for recurrent parental disorder.

Whilst this has invited genetic interpretations around heritability to children, it is also evident that the environmental conditions are a major factor (Jaffee, Caspi, Moffitt, Polo-Tomás, & Taylor, 2007). Indeed, the transmission of risk from parent to child also occurs where the carer is a stepparent and across different types of disorder, for example, from parental alcoholism to offspring depression (Jacobs & Wolin, 1989). It appears that the chronicity and severity of impairment resulting from parental disorder is the more critical factor. Also, studies show that although father's clinical diagnoses exert weaker effects than the mother's, the presence of two psychiatrically ill parents substantially increases likelihood of disorder in the offspring (Ramchandani & Stein, 2003). Since individuals with depression have a higher likelihood of being partnered by those with psychiatric disorder, this increases the likelihood of two parents being affected intergenerationally. Thus, 25% of husbands of women with depression have been shown to have disorders themselves, and as many as 41% of wives of men with a psychiatric diagnosis were similarly affected. This is argued to be not only through 'assortative pairing', whereby individuals with disorder appear to select partners with similar impairment, but also through the subsequent development of disorder in the partner of an affected individual due to relationship problems arising. The resulting impeded parenting style and related adversity can impact on the child and its development and create vulnerability and risk for future depression (Weissman, Gammon, John, Merikangas et al., 1987).

The accumulating effects of adverse environments in childhood on health outcomes have been well documented. Thus, early investigation by Michael Rutter and his team, of a cumulative index of the number of stressors required for disorder to occur led to his conceptualisation of resilience, with a single or lower number of factors being protective (Rutter, 1985b), whilst a higher score increases disorder risk, repeated in other similar investigations (Jaffee et al., 2007). However, before examining such dose effects of childhood adversity on adult disorder, it is first necessary to consider types and definitions of childhood adversity further and to include child maltreatment in the form of neglect and abuse as a vulnerability factor for adult disorder.

Childhood maltreatment and trauma

As described in the previous section, investigating adverse single experiences in childhood, such as loss of mother, showed that the loss itself was subsidiary to any poor parental care received before or after the loss (Harris, Brown, & Bifulco, 1986). Further investigation showed that not only childhood neglect but also physical abuse and antipathy (Bifulco, Brown, & Harris, 1994), sexual abuse (Bifulco, Brown, & Adler, 1991) and psychological abuse (Bifulco, Moran, Baines, Bunn, & Stanford, 2003) substantially contributed to risk of adult depression. However, these experiences only increased risk when they were at 'marked' or 'moderate' levels of severity rather than mild levels. Those at 'marked' severity were also likely to constitute trauma experiences defined in terms of risk to life and sexual violence (Larsen & Berenbaum, 2017). Therefore, the investigation of childhood neglect/ abuse moves the model away from general deprivation to that of more personally targeted and potentially traumatic childhood experience. Whilst early studies tended to focus on these experiences individually, more recent investigation utilises combined indices of these. This works most effectively when similar severity levels and scoring can be applied across the different experiences, following the same methods used in life events severity categorisation (Bifulco & Moran, 1998).

As shown in Chapter 3, trauma events have particular and more extensive impacts than other severe life events, including dissociation, poor emotional regulation and memory disturbance when not effectively processed. These include a range of PTSD outcomes (van der Kolk, Pelcovitz, Roth, Mandel et al., 1996). The diagnosis of complex PTSD sometimes occurs, whereby the early trauma experience itself becomes part of the diagnosis including developmental trauma and other co-morbid disorders (van der Kolk, 2001). This includes abusive experience in childhood from parents or carers or other adults. Abused children frequently can't seek help due to the secrecy imposed and the barriers to telling others (e.g. reprisals, stigma). The intensity and solitariness of the experience can lead to related psychological problems including dissociation, fragmentary processing of the events and lack of emotional regulation (van der Kolk, 2005). In models of adult vulnerability, childhood and adolescent maltreatment needs to be labelled as distal vulnerability being mediated by later more proximal factors that involve the individual's current psychosocial vulnerability such as insecure attachment style.

Here, we consider dose effects of childhood experience, beginning with general adversity and then specifying findings for maltreatment and trauma experience.

Adverse childhood experiences (ACE) and dose effects

The 'dose' effect whereby each additional adversity increases later disorder incrementally has been made most prominent in the ACE studies by Felitti and colleagues in the USA (Felitti, 2002). This research survey investigated thousands of US health insurance claims of individuals in midlife and found greatly increased illness in those who reported multiples of adversity under the age of 18. They devised the ACE questionnaire[1] which has ten items, five of which cover adverse family circumstances (loss of parent, parental physical and mental illness, parental violence, parental criminality). Another five items cover maltreatment including material neglect, emotional neglect, physical abuse, sexual abuse and emotional abuse to the child. Each item has a 'yes' or 'no' response. A total score of four or more on the questionnaire was associated with greatly increased risk of psychological disorder and also physical health outcomes (such as cardio-vascular disorder and diabetes) (Dong et al., 2004; Felitti et al., 1998). A gradient was observed between number of items and later life disorder, thus indicating a dose effect.

These effects are impressive, not least because of the focus on physical health as well as mental health outcomes in midlife, and have largely been replicated (Nanni, Uher, & Danese, 2012). However, the questionnaire utilised is minimal, and given recent criticism of such brief retrospective measures (Bifulco & Schimmenti, 2019), more robust and intensive approaches need to be utilised to validate findings. The dose effects have also been examined in intensive interview approaches. The CECA (Childhood Experience of Care and Abuse) interview developed in the Bedford Square team has led to extensive work on childhood neglect/abuse and adversity in the Brown and Harris tradition and is outlined here.

The CECA[2] is a retrospective and intensive interview of childhood and adolescence which covers a wide range of experience – both family circumstance and maltreatment – in a chronological scheme from birth to the end of the 16th year of life (Bifulco & Moran, 1998). It can be used with adolescents, adults and those in older age (Bifulco, Jacobs, Oskis, Cavana, & Spence, 2019). It was developed with probing interview questions to evoke a similar narrative to the LEDS interview, with investigator rather than self-reported judgements. It also provided careful coverage of repeat occurrences of maltreatment and adversity in different settings or by different perpetrators in a time frame. The interview has tested reliability and has been validated extensively in a hundred pairs of sisters (Bifulco, Brown, Lillie, & Jarvis, 1997). It is also validated internationally (Gianonne et al., 2011; Harkness & Wildes, 2002; Kaess et al., 2011). This interview is able to establish a full account of childhood experience as well as to quantify the type and severity of childhood neglect and abuse experiences in relation to adult depression. Figure 4.4 shows CECA maltreatment definitions.

The CECA provides a detailed definition for each type of neglect or abuse and information for the correct reliable scoring of severity on a 4-point scale. This is for the investigator to make objective judgements in assessing the severity of each abuse, over and above the participants' subjective account and response. Thus, each experience is rated as more or less severe, and are repeated for change over time and from different perpetrators. In the analysis, the peak severity is utilised for each of the maltreatment experiences as well as relationship to perpetrator. Analysis shows that the more severe the experience, the higher the rate of both lifetime and 12-month depression (Bifulco & Moran, 1998). Thus, for example, in the sample of 303 London women (see studies 5 and 6 combined, Appendix 1), neglect showed an increase in depression rate according to severity from 28, 38, 51 to 66% for the ratings of 'none', 'some', 'moderate' and 'marked' levels of neglect. For physical abuse, the rates were 22, 26, 36 and 50%, respectively. This dose effect confirms other findings but also shows that the mild levels of neglect or abuse do not have long-lasting effect. For subsequent analyses, only 'marked' or 'moderate' scores (severe neglect or abuse) were utilised in indices. An index

---

CECA neglect and abuse definitions (Bifulco & Moran, 1998)

Antipathy – cold or critical parenting. Instances include critical comments, angry hostile interaction, scapegoating and rejection. This is sometimes considered emotional abuse.

Neglect – indifference to the child's physical, material and emotional needs in domains of feeding, clothing, hygiene, medical care, education, friendships and sympathetic support.

Physical abuse – attacks on the child which have the potential for harm. Severity determined by frequency, chronicity and intensity of attack.

Sexual abuse – inappropriate sexual contact or solicitation by adult or older peer, either related or non-related. Severity determined by extent of sexual contact, power exerted and closeness of prior relationship.

Psychological abuse – coercive control exerted through psychological or emotional means to confuse, disorientate and create submissiveness. It covers a range of techniques including dehumanisation, terrorising, emotional blackmail, deprivation of basic needs and valued objects. Severity determined by intensity, chronicity and range of strategies used.

Figure 4.4 CECA maltreatment definitions.

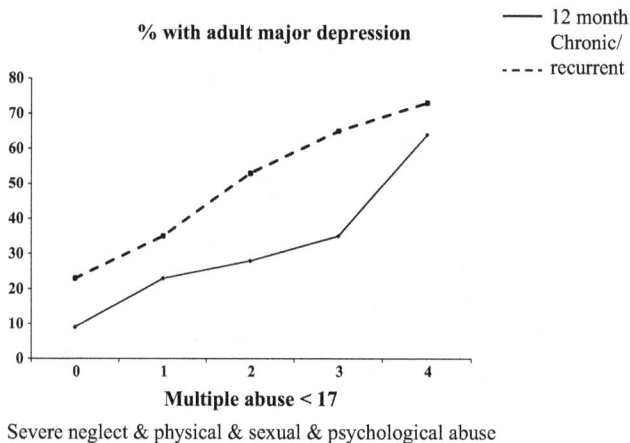

Figure 4.5 Dose effects of childhood maltreatment on adult depression. (303 midlife women – Coping and Sisters combined).

of severe neglect or physical abuse or sexual abuse or psychological abuse raised the risk of depression three-fold in adults (Bifulco & Moran, 1998) and five-fold in adolescents for any disorder (Bifulco et al., 2002). A dose effect was evident with the multiples of experience increasing rates of depression (see Figure 4.5).

However, other adversity indices such as loss of parent or parental conflict had low or no association with later life depression and showed no evidence of dose effects using the CECA. The odds ratio (OR) in the Sisters series for depression showed no significant findings in relation to loss of parent (OR = 1.0), parental psychiatric illness (OR = 1.2), parental alcoholism (OR = 1.1) or parental physical illness (OR = 1.3). Therefore, neglect or abuse to the child has substantially more impact than the family context aspects in this study. However, the family context variables (loss of parent, parental alcoholism or illness) were shown to increase the family risk of child maltreatment (i.e. neglect or abuse) three-fold (Bifulco & Moran, 1998).

As well as dose effects, there was also evidence of specificity of effects. In this instance, a single type of severe abuse was shown to be sufficient to indicate high disorder risk. For example, using the CECA in a representative London adolescent sample demonstrated severe sexual abuse had a 7.8-fold increase in behavioural or emotional disorder being present compared with physical abuse from mother showing a 3.7-fold increase (Bifulco et al., 2002). Similarly, when replicating findings in another high-risk London adolescent sample, there was an OR of 8.8 for maternal neglect in relation to deliberate self-harm and 3.7 for her maternal physical abuse (Bifulco et al., 2014), indicating a higher association of neglect with self-harm. Thus, it can be seen that patterning is possible for individual types of childhood maltreatment and disorder, and this can vary by type of disorder and life stage of the individual. So, any one abusive experience can be of importance clinically, not only multiple experiences.

This intricate relationship of childhood maltreatment (neglect, physical abuse, sexual abuse or psychological abuse), as measured by the CECA, to adult depression has been established (Bifulco et al., 1987, 1994, 2003) over repeated samples and confirmed in meta-analytic study (Infurna et al., 2016). Its relationship to adolescent disorder is confirmed for emotional disorder (Schimmenti & Bifulco, 2015) as well as behavioural disorder (Bifulco et al., 2002), deliberate self-harm (Bifulco et al., 2014; Kaess et al., 2011) and for schizotypal characteristics (Sheinbaum et al., 2015). The impacts of such neglect or abuse on clinical disorder are thus substantial and wide ranging.

As well as these objective indicators of childhood neglect and abuse, there are feeling states associated with such maltreatment which are important. Those tested include childhood feelings of helplessness, worthlessness, hopelessness and shame (Bifulco & Moran, 1998; Harris, Brown, & Bifulco, 1990; Spence et al., 2019). Other responses involve anger, violence and disruptive behaviour (Kazemian, Widom, & Farrington, 2011; Widom & Ames, 1994). In general, childhood neglect and abuse has been associated with intensified negative affect and greater decreases in positive affect during subsequent daily events with reduced feelings of mastery (Infurna, Rivers, Reich, & Zautra, 2015).

Continuities of adversity into adulthood

It is important to consider the mechanisms whereby childhood adverse experiences result in greater adult adversity, later severe life events and clinical disorder.

Whilst initial research showed links of childhood adversity to particular demographic risks such as teenage pregnancy and lower socio-economic status (Harris et al., 1987), more extensive investigation examined stressors more widely across the adult life course using the Adult Life Phase Interview (ALPHI) (Bifulco, Bernazzani, Moran, & Ball, 2000). The ALPHI assessed the severity of chronic adversity in each of five domains (partnership, parenthood, social arena, material sphere and miscellaneous domain) and within determined life phases and linked change points. This is akin to a shortened and elongated LEDS interview with a focus on the severity of chronic stressors or long-term problems. An index was produced summing the presence of a high level of adversity (marked or moderate) in each domain or change point over all the life phases. Results showed that this index of high adult lifetime adversity added to models of depression in addition to childhood adversity (Bifulco et al., 2000). This also contributed in separate analyses to the likelihood of domestic violence (Bifulco, Damiani, et al., 2019); here, a dose effect was evident with the higher the number of adult adversities, the higher the likelihood of partner violence occurring (see Figure 4.6B).

The adult adversity index also contributed to financial difficulties (Spence et al., 2019) and impacts in older age (Bifulco, Jacobs, et al., 2019). When childhood neglect or abuse was examined in relation to such adult adversity, a further dose effect for recurrent adult depression was found.

When the specific example of adult-partner violence was examined, this was found to be associated with lower social class, single-parent status and childhood neglect/abuse but not to ethnicity (Bifulco, Damiani, et al., 2019). Another dose effect was evident, with the more childhood adversity an individual experienced, the greater the likelihood of parental violence occurring (Bifulco, Damiani, et al., 2019) (see Figure 4.6A). Interestingly, there was no association of physical abuse in childhood and increased risk of partner violence indicative of

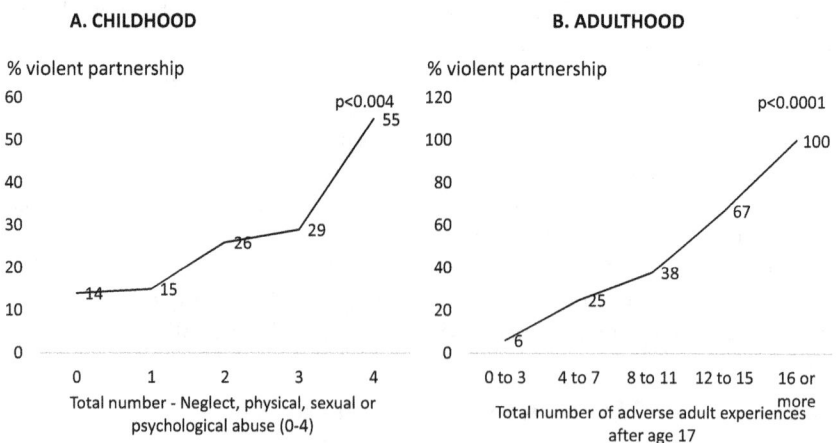

Figure 4.6 Dose effects: adversity and partner violence.

aberrant learning patterns or cycle of physical violence. Neglect in childhood had a particularly strong relationship with adult partner violence and this replicated earlier research (Andrews & Brown, 1988). Psychological abuse also played an important role (LoCascio et al., 2018) (see Figure 4.6).

When childhood adversity was examined prospectively in a representative sample of women in relation to severe life events in the 12 months before interview, a significant relationship was found – with a doubling of risk of experiencing a severe event among individuals with childhood neglect or abuse (Bifulco et al., 1987). Among a sample of women selected for having proximal vulnerability (NES or NECR), childhood adversity was found in 58% of the sample, significantly higher than the 29% in the representative one (Bifulco et al., 1998) (sample 5, Appendix 1).

Childhood maltreatment and psychological vulnerability

As indicated earlier, childhood maltreatment relates to problems in attachment style in adolescence and later life. Thus, experiences of neglect or abuse in childhood or teenage years doubled the risk of insecure attachment style in adulthood (Bifulco et al., 2002). Evidence was also shown of specific associations, with neglect/emotional abuse relating to anxious attachment style and physical or sexual abuse to angry-dismissive style (Bifulco & Thomas, 2012). As already described, insecure attachment style is shown to mediate with both anxiety and depression – the styles most implicated are those fearful and angry-dismissive. Both of these also relate to anxiety states (social anxiety and generalised anxiety disorder, respectively) (Bifulco et al., 2006).

Childhood adversity also related to cognitive distortions of low self-esteem, with NES associated with neglect/emotional abuse (lack of care) (Brown et al., 1990a; Brown, Bifulco, Veiel, et al., 1990). Such early experience was associated with double the rate of NES in adulthood. However, a path analysis model showed that early neglect is a more important predictor of the index of negative relationships (NECR), and these together predict NES, with lack of care associated with a fourfold rate of NECR.

Thus, childhood experiences of neglect or abuse can be seen to link with proximal vulnerability factors of problem-relating styles as well as low self-esteem.

Having indicated how a social and psychological pathway linking adverse environments can emanate from childhood adverse experiences, we will now outline biological impacts also related to early life experience.

Biological impacts of childhood adversity

Early life adversity is associated with biological risk which can create alternative pathways to depression or other poor health outcomes. Adverse childhood experience relates to a range of biological changes in the child that can impede development and future coping with stress (McCrory et al., 2012). Differences at the neurobiological level may represent adaptations to early experiences of heightened stress that lead to an increased risk of disorder. The elements of biological change thought to be directly affected by childhood maltreatment are neuroendocrine changes associated with cortisol (stress hormone) and structural and functional brain differences as well as genes influencing sensitivity to adversity. These will be outlined below.

The Hypothalamic–Pituitary–Adrenal (HPA) axis represents one of the body's core stress response systems. This comprises the hypothalamus, pituitary gland and adrenal glands which play a pivotal role in triggering the stress response by releasing certain chemicals, such as adrenocorticotropic hormone (ACTH) and cortisol. Thus, the HPA axis rouses the body for action when it's faced with a stressor. Exposure to stress triggers release of corticotrophin-releasing hormone (CRH) and arginine vasopressin (AVP) from the paraventricular nucleus of the hypothalamus, which in turn stimulate secretion of ACTH that acts on the adrenal cortex to synthesise cortisol. Feedback loops at several levels ensure that the system is returned to homeostasis since chronically elevated cortisol levels can have deleterious effects on health (Gunnar & Quevedo, 2007). Levels of cortisol have sudden increases under stress, together with adrenaline and usually these then decrease when the stressor is managed (Loveday, 2016). The body can also maintain a level of high alert when stressors are chronic. When this occurs in childhood, it can increase dysregulation in adulthood and have deleterious impacts on health, including the immune system and memory function due to toxic effects on the hippocampus. It is also implicated in risk for depression (Harris et al., 2000), and patients with depression exhibit both decreased brain serotonin function and increased cortisol secretion (Cowen, 2002). However, the evidence of salivary cortisol levels in those depressed is inconsistent, as is that of depleted serotonin, casting some doubt over these associations (Cowen, 2002).

Alterations in the HPA axis activity (as measured by salivary cortisol activity) have been observed in children following a range of adverse early life experiences (Fisher, Stoolmiller, Gunnar, & Burraston, 2007). For example, atypical patterns of HPA axis activity have been reported in children who experienced the early loss of a caregiver (Meinlschmidt & Heim, 2005), in children who were maltreated in their family of origin (De Bellis et al., 1999) and in children who were subjected to severe neglect as a result of institutional rearing in developing countries (Carlson & Earls, 1997). The characteristic pattern of alterations noted for these children is a flattening of diurnal (morning-to-evening) cortisol activity, owing largely to low early morning cortisol levels (Gunnar & Vazquez, 2001). Similar patterns associated with chronic stress have been noted in adults (Heim, Ehlert, & Hellhammer, 2000), and it is presumed that these flattened or hypoactive patterns reflect downregulation of the HPA axis following periods of heightened activity early in life.

The argument has been put forward that traumatised children initially exhibit complex developmental disorders which are environmentally induced but which later branch towards more specific disorders such as depression and anxiety (Cicchetti, 1996). However, the data on the stress physiology of abused children can be challenging to interpret (Gunnar & Quevedo, 2007) with concurrent disorder contributing to the presentation of stress functioning. For example, maltreated boys at a summer camp who had interalising (emotional) disorder had higher cortisol levels than non-maltreated boys or those with externalising (behavioural) disorder (Cicchetti & Rogosch, 2001). In a study of maltreated preschool-aged children and socioeconomic status-matched controls, maltreated children exhibited less cortisol reactivity and produced even lower cortisol levels on days when there were high levels of conflict and aggression in their classrooms (Hart, Gunnar, & Cicchetti, 1995).

McCrory and colleagues have undertaken two influential reviews of the impact of childhood maltreatment on neurobiological mechanisms (McCrory et al., 2012; McCrory, Gerin, & Viding, 2017). In the first, they outline the association of childhood maltreatment on neuroendocrine function as well as structural and functional differences at the level of the brain. These can influence the neurobiological circuitry underpinning psychological and emotional development (McCrory et al., 2012). Specifically, the review identifies atypical development of the HPA axis, the core stress response systems as associated with childhood maltreatment in line with that outlined above. They identify studies which support that early stress can lead to an ongoing dysregulation of the HPA axis which predisposes to psychiatric vulnerability. In fact, they note that chronically elevated cortisol levels have generally deleterious impacts on health.

In terms of structural brain impacts, McCrory and colleagues identify problems in the development of the hippocampus by childhood maltreatment. The hippocampus plays a central role in learning and memory, functions impaired when exposed to chronic stress. For example, adults with PTSD and childhood maltreatment are shown to have smaller hippocampal volumes. Other cortical structures include the prefrontal cortex which plays a major role in regulating cognitive and emotional processes, with smaller prefrontal cortex volume, less prefrontal white matter and larger grey matter evident among those with maltreatment. Finally, the corpus callosum – which is the largest white matter structure in the brain and controls processes including arousal, emotional and higher cognitive abilities – is also shown to be decreased in volume in those maltreated.

Their second review looks specifically at functional brain imaging studies and the amygdala in relation to latent vulnerability (McCrory et al., 2017). By latent vulnerability, they mean neurobiological changes that, whilst they increase likelihood of clinical disorder, can exist even without disorder occurring. The brain imaging studies show that the amygdala, which plays a central role in evaluating threat and fear conditioning, can be either heightened or lowered as neural responsiveness in maltreated samples. Another aspect is the blunting of neural response to anticipation and receipt of rewards and other emotional regulation. Thus, there is growing evidence of direct impact of maltreatment on brain and neurobiological development which can impact on aspects of cognitive and emotional development and fear responses to increase risk of clinical disorder.

Furthermore, there is growing evidence for insecure attachment style, emanating from childhood adversity, to be associated with HPA response and high levels of cortisol. Thus, a study of married couples (Jaremka et al., 2013) and of school girls (Oskis, Loveday, Hucklebridge, Thorn, & Clow, 2010) showed anxious attachment styles in particular related to raised rates in salivary cortisol. Adults with insecure attachment style or with lower levels of maternal warmth have also shown greater increases in cortisol throughout the day than their counterparts with secure attachment (Jaremka et al., 2013; Lucas-Thompson & Granger, 2014). It is argued that this emanates from childhood where relationships with parents can influence emotional states as well as the associated biological functions. It is likely therefore that individuals with insecure attachment style may experience heightened stress generally and even in response to positive life events.

Thus, it appears that adverse early experiences produce different patterns of stress responding in different individuals; hyperreactivity in some and seemingly hyporeactivity in others. Although the nature and timing of adverse or maltreating experience may partly explain these differences, it is likely that to some extent they also reflect individual differences that have a genetic contribution.

The serotonin transporter gene and childhood adversity

Studies of the interaction of the serotonin transporter genotype and environment upon adult depression have also examined distal vulnerability factors and shown childhood maltreatment to play a significant role in the genesis of disorder (Caspi et al., 2003; Fisher et al., 2013). However, the type of depression (i.e. that chronic rather than acute) is argued to influence results in a study undertaken by Brown and colleagues which showed that the short allele version of 5-HTTLPR moderated the relationship between childhood neglect or abuse and *chronic* depression in adulthood but not new *acute* depressive onsets (Brown et al., 2013). With this prospective study, the researchers were also able to examine effects on new acute onsets of disorder. They found that the G × E interaction associated with childhood maltreatment played a stronger role than that for G × E with severe life events occurring close to onset. They argue that childhood maltreatment is associated with a particularly high risk of an adult depression taking a chronic course (i.e. lasting 12 months or more), and this explains the link. They found that 5-HTTLPR did not moderate the effects of either childhood maltreatment or severe life events on new acute depressive onsets. They conclude that the short variant of the serotonin transporter gene specifically sensitises to the effect of early-life experience of neglect/abuse on whether an adult depressive episode takes a chronic course. This interaction may be responsible for a substantial proportion of cases of chronic depression in the general population (Brown, Adler, & Bifulco, 1988).

Differential genetic susceptibility

One intriguing development to have emerged from studies of gene–environment interaction is the model of differential susceptibility (Belsky et al., 2009). This constitutes an alternative to the vulnerability-provoking agent model (Bakermans-Kranenburg & IJzendoorn, 2007). It states that individuals vary in their developmental plasticity, with more plastic or malleable individuals (designated 'orchids') more susceptible than others (designated as 'daisies') to environmental influences in a far-better-or-far-worse manner. That is, they are more sensitised to *both* negative and supportive environments with either adverse or positive developmental sequelae, respectively (Belsky et al., 2007). Thus, a proportion of individuals (those less malleable or daisies) may be less affected by adversity in childhood. The others (those more malleable or orchids) will be more sensitive to their environment and will suffer more if exposed to inadequacies of care and problem parenting, but flourish to a greater degree in benign circumstances. The 'daisies' will be hardier and less impacted by either harsh or benign environments. The seven-repeat allele of the DRD4 gene has attracted particular attention in supporting this hypothesis as well as the 'short' 5-HTT promoter region allele with children having the gene variants showing more negative and positive outcomes depending on the quality of maternal caregiving (Bakermans-Kranenburg & van Ijzendoorn, 2006).

Thus, it is argued that the genetic contribution which makes children do poorly under harsh conditions can also make them flourish under benign conditions. This is an interesting example of how genetic influence varies under environmental conditions. This model needs further investigation, for example, to show that even with a very high level of childhood adversity involving multiple neglect and abuse, the less malleable group (i.e. daisies) do indeed remain impervious to its impact. Given direct impact of high levels of adversity on brain development and the HPA axis (McCrory, De Brito, & Viding, 2010), this model may not hold under all conditions. It does however provide an interesting variant on the vulnerability model and has enormous implications for intervention for those with more malleable predispositions.

Clinical implications

Vulnerability to psychological disorder is key to understanding differential stress responses to severe life events. For adults, this requires a lifespan perspective and implicates damage to early child development as a precursor of poor lifetime health. Key elements of childhood adversity comprise social disadvantage which causes stress for families including children and can impair parenting which lead to further trajectories of negative environmental stressors longer term. Maltreatment encompasses childhood trauma experience (in the form of neglect or abuse) not only from parent figures but also from other predators (specifically for sexual abuse) and greatly increases the risk of clinical disorder, with highest rates in adolescence but also extending into adulthood and even older age. Both types of adversity (social and trauma) show dose effects in relating to later adult adversity and emotional disorder. However, for the more traumatic maltreatment experiences, even single experiences of severe neglect or abuse are significant and can be damaging with some patterning of type of single trauma to type of disorder. These are important messages for clinicians.

There is some evidence that genetic inheritance may moderate intervention efficacy (Belsky & van Ijzendoorn, 2015). Biological approaches to vulnerability may therefore affect treatment in actionable ways (Belsky & Van Ijzendoorn, 2015). The G × I (gene × intervention approach) advocates a personalised approach to intervention efficacy in terms of 'what works for whom'. This could potentially identify in terms of a genetic profile, individuals who would be most receptive to particular types of therapy, and also those with more genetically influenced resilience. The research indicating genetic difference in hardiness/sensitivity indicates differential impact of adversity. Thus, identifying sensitivity might be relevant to early interventions. Alternatively, it may be that this research has greater input into explaining resilience.

Some therapies (such as psychodynamic) focus specifically on childhood experience and memories of that experience in attempting to work through the unlocked residual trauma, that is, distal vulnerability factors. Other approaches such as CBT attempt to work on the negative cognitive-affective responses which endure into adulthood or proximal vulnerability factors. Their claim is that such change can be affected without requiring exploration of childhood memories. Others such as solution-focused therapies draw on clients' perceptions of what works for them personally in dealing with adversity and stressors. Similar to CBT, they do not require detailed exploration of childhood experiences, but instead involve exploration of resources and approaches that work in their current situations. That is, a focus on proximal vulnerability and recent severe life events.

Therapists view their clients' current beliefs, feelings and behaviours as needing to be re-aligned for a more positive and adaptive outlook. This work can be aided by increased support in the natural environment to influence more positive coping. This is how individuals can cope successfully with stressful life events and will be discussed further in Chapter 8. Interventions need to focus on vulnerability or ways of overcoming vulnerabilities, and to date, these have mainly utilised the psychological strand in the model outlined earlier. This is because in order to utilise support and help from services, individuals need to be able to trust sufficiently and once engaged to be able to admit need and disclose problems and concerns. This is difficult for those with insecure attachment styles. Such a step also requires the confidence of feelings of self-worth – that the client feels worthy of support, help and care. Individual's attachment styles are very amenable to therapeutic intervention. For example, psychotherapy works on issues such as trust in the therapist as central to change. Also, the content of therapy can examine cognitive-affective barriers to closeness, fear or anger linked to social interaction. This can be extended to couples' therapy and to family therapy to understand interpersonal relationships better. Interpersonal therapy is also a candidate for effecting positive changes in communication and conflict resolution in relationships to allow for improved attachment behaviour. However, it needs to be understood that proximal vulnerability can create barriers to individuals in need ever engaging with services in the first place. Thus, earlier community interventions are also needed.

A focus on vulnerability allows for interventions and early prevention work to be undertaken since it is a more enduring phenomenon than severe life events themselves. With their origins in childhood experience, it makes sense for interventions to occur in early years where possible. This was highlighted in Marmot's review of preventative work in healthcare nationally which in concluding focused on the first five years of life (Marmot, 2020). Whilst this has led to 'Early Years' projects in schools, children's centres and the health service, it has fallen by the wayside during austerity[3] despite parallel policy reviews seeking greater mental health provision in schools[4] (Davidson & Bifulco, 2018). However, there is recent policy around Mental Health Support Teams that are now in schools with some promising early work being done.[5] This in combination with a national focus on safeguarding issues in children and adolescents should aim to reduce the harms arising from maltreatment. With additional therapeutic support for survivors of childhood maltreatment, the conditions for being susceptible to repeat episodes of emotional disorder would thus be reduced.

Notes

1 http://traumadissociation.com/ace
2 https://lifespantraining.org.uk/types-of-training/childhood-experience-of-care-abuse-ceca/ceca-introduction-and-background/
3 https://www.theguardian.com/society/2018/apr/05/1000-sure-start-childrens-centres-may-have-shut-since-2010
4 https://www.gov.uk/government/publications/mental-health-and-wellbeing-provision-in-schools
5 https://www.england.nhs.uk/mental-health/cyp/trailblazers/

Section 2

Life event measurement

5 Contending with atheoretical measurement

We have presented a model of life events that is anchored in the Life Events and Difficulties Schedule (LEDS) tradition of eliciting narrative accounts about experience in context. However, in practice, much of the richness that comes from collecting this sort of in-depth contextual description has been lost to both psychology and psychiatry through the increased use of checklist self-report tools. This is understandable in economic terms given the greater expense in time and trained research staff required for interview approaches. Interviews are deemed impractical for large-scale research projects particularly in the newer areas of genetics where vast numbers of participants are needed. Due to these and other factors, life events' checklists have re-emerged in clinical research and the use of interviews declined.

However, checklist methodologies cannot capture the nuances implicated within more sophisticated models of life events as discussed in this book and potentially vastly underestimate the number and severity of stressors. From our previous discussion, it should now be clear that life events have an impact not only due to the life event per se but also due to what that particular life event represents for the individual in their life context and how any underlying vulnerability is triggered. This chapter will provide a brief overview of the numerous methodological flaws of checklists and outline some of the consequences resulting from their continued dominance. Whilst some of this may be obvious at this point following earlier chapters, identifying these helps us to bear in mind the real significance and meaning behind life events. We will also describe some of the ways in which researchers have tried to improve on checklists to achieve at least some of the benefits of spoken questioning.

Methodological problems with checklists

There are numerous papers on the subject of life events measurement spanning many decades, these continuing to the present day (Brown, Sklair, Harris, & Birley, 1973; Dohrenwend, 2006; Gorman & Brown, 1992; Harkness & Monroe, 2016; Slavich, Stewart, Esposito, Shields, & Auerbach, 2019). One would expect the literature to constantly evolve, where the earlier concerns are resolved as new issues arise. Unfortunately, often historical concerns and the arguments made remain principally unchanged as the research literature moves onto other topics. The life event literature has, however, remained consistent in showing that life event checklists have a number of methodological flaws and are limited in their capacity for measuring anything meaningful. Below, we list some of the major limitations that have been levelled at checklists and their use.

- **Static list of events**

    Checklists cannot include all the possible types of events that can be experienced. Indeed, by their very design, they have a limited number of items and therefore inevitably have to focus on a few. Whilst some have selected their items from events identified as severe by interview (e.g. Brugha, Bebbington, Tennant, & Hurry, 1985), these are likely to change for different samples and over time. The types of event experienced by people are dynamic – when checklists were developed in the 1960s who could have imagined the internet, IVF treatment, climate change and an increasingly globalised world? Events such as online harm through trolling or failure of a final IVF course for a much-wanted pregnancy or frequency of flooding or even Covid-19 and its lockdown would simply not appear.

- **Lack of context**

    One of the main criticisms levelled at life events checklists is the lack of context to specify the likely meaning of the event for the individual. Although checklists may contain some specificity (e.g. serious illness of close family member: mother, father, etc.), most only involve a brief description of the event in question (e.g. death, divorce, pregnancy) but otherwise give no specific information. As we have argued, context is key to understanding the impact of any given event and to assume that all individuals will be expected to experience the same level of impact given the same brief event summary, contains a number of presumptions. For example, ticking 'pregnancy' tells you nothing about the individual's planning regarding parenthood, their health or financial security and partnership arrangements. Of all events, this is one which can elicit the broadest range of responses given different circumstances. Similarly, checking 'divorce' as occurring does not give details of whether it was amicable, costly or enforced.

- **Assumption of shared ideas**

    The researcher and respondent might have vastly different ideas about what constitutes a certain type of event. For instance, being diagnosed with a 'serious illness' might seem straightforward but is there universal agreement as to what constitutes serious? For example, would everyone agree that type II diabetes or arthritis is serious? Another example is a 'major change in financial state,' what is major? £500, £5000 or £50,000? If the respondent is already very wealthy, perhaps none; if they are struggling to make ends meet; perhaps all. Once an answer is ticked on the checklist, we have no further validational information as to what occurred.

- **Compound questions**

    A good example of an item that may seem like a single question but actually contains two is: 'have you or your partner been sacked from your job or been made redundant?' The implications around being sacked are different to those of redundancy. Being sacked suggests some wrongdoing and potential for shame or humiliation (for a discussion of the importance of humiliation, see Chapter 2), whereas redundancy suggests that it was outside their influence and may, for instance, come with a nice financial package. However, a simple check does not allow us to know which occurred.

- **Multiples of the same event**

  Events may happen more than once in the time period under investigation but most checklists only enable the respondent one opportunity to check the box. Whilst checklists work on a 'dose' effect (producing a total number of events) rather than a specificity effect (the one event which matches the individual's worst nightmare), it underestimates that this given multiples of events in the same category cannot be scored. This ignores the idea that multiples of the same event can compound the stress experienced to induce hopelessness. For example, 'have you or another individual who lives with you suffered a miscarriage or a stillbirth?' It is possible for numerous miscarriages to occur within a year; if the individual is keen to have a child, it is possible that each miscarriage may be experienced as more negative than the last (see Chapter 2 for a discussion of entrapment and D-matching events). Similarly, a person can experience more than one job loss, could move house a number of times or be taken to court on several occasions within any given study time period.

- **Event sequencing**

  Often, numerous events occur within a short time frame as part of a sequence of a situation developing. For example, the following scenario is likely but not easily represented on a checklist: a diagnosis of a serious medical condition and a month later, a complex operation. Does the timing of the two events make a difference to whether a respondent might rate them as one or two events? For instance, if the operation occurred only a day later or three months later? Similarly, do individuals discount certain events in retrospect because they know the outcome? For example, someone who had just received a diagnosis of cancer would probably agree that they have experienced a 'serious' personal illness, but if by the time of completing the questionnaire, they knew the cancer was a mild form and readily treated would they still tick 'yes'? If someone had a baby who died after two months would they agree to two events: gaining a new family member and death of a close family member or would the death eclipse the preceding event?

- **Event dating**

  One of the main reasons that life events have been so extensively studied is due to their temporal relationship with psychological disorder. Many studies have shown that onset is usually within 3–6 months of the triggering event. However, although many questionnaires ask about life events occurring within the last year, they do not ask for precise dating of any given event, including those occurring during or after the depression. It is also impossible to check whether the respondent is accurately reporting that the event happened in the past 12 months. A similar issue arises with symptom checklist scales that onset of disorder cannot be determined and thus sequences of event and disorder not established.

- **Chronic problems**

    Life events are discrete events that happen over a short period of time, whereas more chronic problems or difficulties are of at least four weeks duration and usually many months long. Checklists do not provide us with the certainty that when respondents are endorsing items, these are definitely acute life events rather than ongoing problems. This can lead to inflated scores because two different concepts (life events and ongoing problems) are reflected together.

- **Stressor/response confusion**

    Many checklists mix up the response with the stressor. For example, changes in eating or sleeping habits are included in some checklists, but can often be the behaviour change resulting from experiencing something stressful or indeed depression. Another example, sexual difficulties, is common in those with depression and other mental health problems and therefore could also be an outcome rather than a cause of psychological distress. Events need to be located as much as possible in external circumstances.

- **Independence**

    There is much debate on the importance of the independence of events which are those that arise from an individual's own behaviour reflective of vulnerability (e.g. frequent arguments or altercations) or indeed from the clinical disorder itself (e.g. lack of concentration leading to accidents). However, it is often not possible to determine from a checklist the extent to which an event is independent of a respondent's intentional action. For example, endorsing 'son or daughter leaving home' may reflect the respondent's child moving out for a job or university study, but it could equally be due to arguments in the household or that the respondent threw his or her child out of the house.

Below, we will use a case study from a recorded LEDS interview undertaken as part of the recent CLEAR study to demonstrate firsthand how the same events were rated (or not) using the LTE-Q checklist severe life event measure. It is also hoped that this will begin to illustrate how interviews are able to gather much more pertinent information and give a fuller understanding of the respondent's experienced life events and a potentially more accurate level of external stressors. This will seek to rebalance the impact in a depression model between the severe life event and underlying vulnerability. This may be important also for resilience models where a large amount of external stress is managed without a depression outcome.

Case examples comparing LEDs and LTE-Q checklist

Two cases will be used to illustrate different levels of overlap between the LEDS reported events and those checked on the LTE-Q checklist. In both these examples, there were difficulties that made the events more challenging. In these particular cases, there was no onset of depression.

Jane's events

A 69-year-old divorced and widowed female, Jane, lives alone in a one-bedroom flat and has a prior history of depression but no symptoms during the study year. She has one friend nearby but no family close. She has a number of health-related difficulties identified by the LEDS which have been going on at least 18 months, some longer. She was diagnosed with epilepsy around a year ago and had been having fits for around four years prior to the diagnosis. It is mostly controlled now but she can still have a few fits a month which lead to accidents, one of which she has had in the past year where she hurt her leg and had to go to the hospital emergency department. Another fit occurred before the study period and resulted in a broken arm which has not healed successfully. Jane also suffers from angina and had a mild heart attack around 18–24 months ago when her cat died. She also suffers from back problems which limits her mobility. These difficulties were not of course rated on the LTE-Q as expected since they are longer term and not acute events.

The LEDS recorded four events for Jane in the past 12 months; the only two severe ones (noted below) were both health-related:

1   An operation on Jane's arm was to correct a previous break two years earlier. It had never healed properly and needed further surgery. She had restricted use of it, and a year earlier had also broken the other arm during an epileptic fit. The operation lasted 3.5 hours and she was told that the surgical intervention would take 6–12 months to heal. Jane had to spend three days in hospital because she had no help at home. After she got home, her neighbours would come in and help her intermittently with things she needed. The doctors were unsure of the prognosis (**LEDS severe event – danger rated; LTE-Q no event rated**).

2   Four months later, Jane's arm had still not healed and was not very functional and she was informed by the doctors that she required a second operation similar to the first. Again, she spent time in hospital because of having no carer and neighbours helping out (**LEDS severe event – danger rated; LTE-Q no event rated**).

Both these events pose a threat to Jane's security and independent living. When she scored the LTE-Q, she endorsed two events: one was a problem with a neighbour, the other the death of a friend. Both had been captured by the LEDS but were non-severe. The LEDS description shows:

3   Problem with a neighbour – Jane was wrongly accused in a phone call to the council of being drunk and shouting and screaming in the lobby of the block of flats where she lives. She believes that it was her neighbour who made the hoax call, when she herself was drunk. Jane confronted her neighbour who

denied it. There was no further outcome although there is a brief difficulty with the neighbour (**LEDS non-severe event; LTE-Q scored event**).

4   Death of a friend: A friend from years ago (Marjorie) dies. Jane was not a confidant, not close and had seen her very infrequently. However, they had been close years earlier. Jane hears of her death through a mutual acquaintance. She does not attend the funeral (**LEDS none-event** – Marjorie was not a close confidant; **LTE-Q event only scored**).

This example shows the LTE-Q failed to pick up the severe health events. Even if Jane had endorsed a 'health' item, she could not have ticked it twice to denote two events. It is not known why Jane did not score these. Therefore, the lack of prompts in the LTE-Q can relate to under-reporting, and the lack of instruction about criteria for which friends are included in severe events also mean that the respondent does not necessarily know which to record. In both instances, Jane reported correctly but not at appropriate severity levels in LEDS terms.

Linda's events

Linda is a 60-year-old married woman living with her husband Sam and adopted son Alfie (aged 29) in a house they own in Kent. Her elderly mother lives in a residential home, and Linda is her carer and visits her weekly. This is despite Linda's own disability due to fibromyalgia.

During the LEDS interview, it transpired that Linda has had five events in the last year, three of which were severe:

1   **Mother's illness deterioration,** December: Her mother aged 95 had dementia (but also a history of psychiatric treatment for anxiety). She had been in a care home for over 20 years with Linda visiting her weekly. The event involved her refusing medication which made her anxiety symptoms recur and made her refuse to eat. Linda was telephoned by the home who were concerned about her mother's health (**LEDS severe event, D-event, danger; LTE-Q scored event**).

2   **Mother died,** February: The funeral was on her 96th birthday (**LEDS severe event, D-event, loss; LTE-Q event scored**).

3   **Husband gave up job,** May: Husband Sam quit his part-time job after a row with the business owners. He was self-employed working in sports centres. This meant they had to be more careful with money, but it did not create financial difficulty. He has other sources of income (**LEDS non-severe event; No LTE-Q event scored**).

4   **House flooded,** June: Serious flooding occurred in the area; this affected Linda's house and covered the whole of the ground floor for more than four hours. Linda was alone in the house unable to leave because she has physical disability die to fibromyalgia. Firemen came and helped move electrical items upstairs. She was able to sleep upstairs. The water abated after four hours but a lot of damage was done to furnishings. Linda was offered a hotel

stay, since her husband and son were away abroad at the time. She refused because she finds hotels difficult to get around due to her disability whereas she has aids at home. When her husband and son returned, she was able to manage. The insurance company has agreed to pay for the damage, but Linda and Sam are having to live with the ruined ground floor. This continues for four months without resolution (**LEDS severe event, danger; LTE-Q scored**).

5   **Row with husband,** June: Linda and her husband have fallen out over managing the flood damage to the house. She would rather move out and get the insurance company to refurbish the property as offered. Her husband wants to stay and do more himself and oversee the refurbishment. This is prolonging the difficult situation since he is making little progress. They have had sharp words and an atmosphere has developed. She can't talk to him easily at present (**LEDS non-severe event; No LTE-Q event scored**).

When the LTE-Q was completed, it successfully identified the following events for Linda – illness of family member, death of family member and one other significant event (not specified but it could be the flood event). However, Linda also had a number of difficulties which were not reflected in the checklist – the 'marked' difficulties involving first the problems caring for her mother which terminated in her death; second those arising from the house flood; and third Linda's own health difficulties with fibromyalgia which cause constant pain and difficult mobility. This latter makes the other issues more difficult to manage given her disability. Thus, what is perhaps interesting about her case is the fact that with this difficulty burden and three severe life events, she did not become depressed therefore implying resilience. This might have been missed with the rated LTE-Q score of '3' which would be fairly low. This case study illustrates a good overlap of the two approaches (interview and checklist) with regard to the severe events, but with minimal information collected in the LTE-Q of context and weighting of events as well as the absence of scoring long-term difficulties, common to all checklist approaches.

Implications for life events research

Despite the many calls for improving life events measurement, life events research goes on essentially unhindered with a great reliance on checklists, with their associated flaws rarely named in study limitations. Indeed, some studies with life events measurement do not even reference what measures they use (e.g. Simhandl, Radua, König, & Amann, 2015), whilst others use measures noted as inspired by the LEDS but without evidence of psychometric properties (Kendler, Karkowski, & Prescott, 1999; Wilhelm et al., 2006). The apparent low regard for life events measurement compared to other variables can be seen in research, for example, when a very comprehensive methodology for genetic analysis is detailed (Wilhelm et al., 2006), but then, little space is given to explaining the life events method, with no details given as to which semi-structured interview was used:

At each follow-up.....all of the participants completed a series of self-report questionnaires in conjunction with a semi-structured interview asking about work and personal life events for each year over the 5-year period. (p. 210) (Wilhelm et al., 2006)

Similarly, in the study by Simhandl and colleagues (2015):

Life events were evaluated *before* and *after* the index episode using the stand-ardized interview and were directly entered in the web-based database. Neg-ative life events were defined as loss of employment, loss/change of residence, end of sentimental relationship, loss of a confidant or family member, acci-dent with admission to hospital, admission to a psychiatric hospital, personal crisis, court case, violence, or all these events experienced by a related per-son (classified as "others"). (p. 167) (Simhandl et al., 2015)

That these researchers give such little attention to life events methodology despite detailed focus on other measures in their model shows the disconnect between research in the field and theoretical papers on the topic. However, the continued use of checklists has real ramifications for the field of life events and research in general. One area that has suffered and continues to suffer due to poor life event measurement techniques is the hugely invested field around gene × environment interactions (as described in Chapter 4).

The LEDS has been compared to checklist measures in a number of stud-ies and has been found to be superior in many ways such as its ability to: pick up both non-severe and severe life events, accurately date events and predict psychological disorder. A comparison of the LEDS and the Psychiatric Epide-miology Research Interview Life Events Scale (PERI) (Dohrenwend, Askenasy, Krasnoff, & Dohrenwend, 1978) found that 62% of the events were misclassified on the PERI as compared to the LEDS (McQuaid, Monroe, Roberts, Kupfer, & Frank, 2000). This was because many events on the PERI were actually ongoing difficulties, some of them outside the established time frame, and others were part of an event that had already been recorded. In another study, the LEDS was compared to the Life Events Checklist for DSM-5 (LEC-5) (Weathers et al., 2013). This is a measure of traumatic events (see Chapter 3) and only captured 32% of severe events found by the LEDS which provoked depression, and it did not provide any dating for the events. In another more detailed study, comparing the LEDS to the LTE-Q (Brugha & Cragg, 1990) in a sample of older adults (Donoghue, Traviss-Turner, House, Lewis, & Gilbody, 2016), the LEDS was su-perior in capturing more severe life events (double the number) and was better able to predict depression.

The above discussion demonstrates that checklists are not as reliable or valid as in-depth interviews. Indeed, a literature review on replication of the original G × E interaction in depression, looking at the candidate gene 5-HTTLPR and life stress (Monroe & Reid, 2008), attributed variable findings to measurement. The review included 12 studies which either replicated or failed to reproduce the original result by Caspi and colleagues (Caspi, Hariri, Holmes, Uher, & Moffitt, 2010). The authors felt that the lack of robust findings was due to both the wide variety of operational definitions used when defining life stress and the resulting methodological approaches employed in measuring it:

> …the majority of studies employed unusual procedures for assessing and operationalising life stress that had no precedent or psychometric justification. Finally, most of the studies were characterised by key methodological and research-design problems (p. 954), (Monroe & Reid, 2008).

It is apparent that checklist questionnaires may lead to life events research failing to replicate extremely important results for psychiatry. This has led researchers to search for other ways in which to collect life events data, which we will outline below.

Beyond checklists and interviews

Whereas the criticisms levelled at checklists tend to be methodological in nature, the critiques of the LEDS are mostly practical. The primary impediment is the length of the process. First, researchers need to be trained in how to use the LEDS and rate the accounts given. Second, the interview itself can take around 45–90 minutes, although if a respondent has had numerous events, this can be longer. Third, rating an interview from the audio recording takes at least two and a half times the length of the interview. (It should be noted that a full transcript is not required, just a summary of each event and difficulty.) Then, with consensus reliability checks for difficult cases, another hour can be added. From start to finish, it is time-intensive for both researchers and participants making large-scale research projects problematic. Nevertheless, there is some evidence that respondents prefer the interview to checklists (Donoghue et al., 2016). A study in which participants completed both the LEDS interview and the LTE-Q showed a clear preference for the interview (op cit). The participants commented that they liked the interview prompts for further information, which allowed them to clarify what had happened. One interviewee stated that they would not have been able to be so honest using the questionnaire. Indeed, some of their concerns by participants echoed the issues raised by researchers around the methodological shortcomings inherent in checklists. For example, they had doubts around the efficacy of the LTE-Q checklist as evidenced by the researchers' qualitative sub-themes stating 'clouds understanding' and 'misses things':

> 'Clouds understanding' refers to the closed responses elicited through the LTE-Q as clouding the understanding of adverse experiences (*'some LTE-Q questions… could be misconstrued,' 'You can tick a box, but it won't put across what you're trying to say…misses the point'*). 'Misses things' relates to the LTE-Q as missing experiences of adversity (*'…doesn't capture my experience and suffering in the same way on the form.'*) (p. 36) (Donoghue et al., 2016)

This suggests that using longer-form and more detailed ways of capturing life event data would not only benefit practitioners but also research respondents. To this end, some have attempted to develop shorter interviews whilst others have attempted to use researcher-led checklists. Anderson and colleagues have termed some of these shorter interviews "second generation" methods of assessing life events/stress (Anderson, Wethington, & Kamarck, 2010). Many of them have sought to shorten the LEDS whilst still maintaining its principles. Being much more comprehensive than checklists, they tend to have good reliability and validity, include the measurement of ongoing difficulties and consider severity ratings for events either by an expert or by the interviewer (Kendler, Walters, et al., 1995; Paykel, 1997; Wilhelm et al., 2006). Some also include panel meetings for agreeing scorings. Although researcher training is still generally required, the main advantage of these types of method is that rating is much quicker. Yet despite this, many of them are not in widespread circulation and have not been used outside the research groups that have developed them (for full comprehensive analysis, see Anderson et al. (2010)). This is perhaps due to the fact that they are based on the LEDS 'gold standard', and if investigators are going to use an interview, they would prefer to use one that is in widespread circulation. Indeed, even in the past decade, many research groups have chosen to use the LEDS with wide-ranging studies, such as assessing persistent depression in women in UK Pakistani women (Chaudhry, Husain, Tomenson, & Creed, 2012) or treatment adherence in individuals with HIV (Bottonari, Safren, McQuaid, Hsiao, & Roberts, 2010) or the relationship between life events and skin cancer (Fagundes et al., 2012).

The alternative method researchers have employed to navigate around some of these pitfalls of checklist measurement is researcher-based versions of checklist. This involves the researcher being present to go through the questionnaire with the respondent. This enables items to be clarified to ensure that the respondent has the same understanding of the checklist as the researchers and confirms the timing of any events. This form of measurement could be particularly important for finding a short but valid method to use in large-scale studies, particularly those looking at interactions between G × E where thousands of participants are required to even hope to look for reasonable effect sizes.

Hosang and colleagues have successfully used an interview-based version of the LTE-Q in several studies of life events and mental health (Hosang, Fisher, Cohen-Woods, McGuffin, & Farmer, 2017; Hosang, Uher, Maugham, McGuffin, & Farmer, 2012). One such study (Hosang et al., 2010) used the interview-based LTE-Q in a large sample of healthy controls and those with either unipolar or bipolar depression. During the questionnaire administration, researchers in the study confirmed events occurred within the relevant time frame and obtained contextual information for the target event to check that it could be rated according to the questionnaire design. They found a significant association between severe life events and depression, concluding that the interview version of the LTE-Q could be suitable for use in such research. However, there was no further validational analysis to verify the events that were accessed through an alternative interview approach.

There is a large literature highlighting the numerous methodological short-comings of checklists, yet despite this, the majority of research studies tend to use them. This reliance on flawed measurement approaches may hamper the ability to find and then replicate significant associations between life events and various outcomes. Interviews have greater reliability and validity, and respondents seem to enjoy them, but they are resource-intensive to the point of being impractical for larger studies. In response to this conundrum, researchers have moved towards measures that are a compromise between checklist and interview methodologies. This includes new online applications which will be outlined in the next chapter.

6 Technology and measuring events

As we have seen from the previous chapter, the methods of capturing life events in a systematic fashion are difficult due to the over-simplicity of questionnaires and the time-consuming and expert knowledge requirement of interview administration. Whilst many other areas of measurement have moved over to digital modes of enquiry, life events have not kept up with the ongoing trend and benefits of such an approach (Spence et al., 2015). This is despite digital advancements in many other areas of psychological research and treatment (Ennis, Sijercic, & Monson, 2018; Schmidt & Wykes, 2012). This chapter will outline the development of an online life events measure that aimed to incorporate some of the benefits of interview approaches. The Computerised Life Events Assessment Record (CLEAR) (Bifulco, Spence, et al., 2019) is one of the first online measures for capturing such complex social stressor assessment. CLEAR synthesises the benefits of online technology with many of the strengths of interviews by directing the user in how to rate severity of life events as well as including difficulties (or long-term problems) in a time-based manner. This is hosted on a dedicated website which includes related questionnaires as well as the life event sections where information is provided through a mixture of checklists for closed responses, text boxes for open-ended responses and logic-driven checklist menus. Futhermore, CLEAR is a dynamic system that uses the data entered to shape what questions are asked and what information is presented to the respondent. We propose that using CLEAR is superior to checklists and less time-consuming than interviews in all aspects (Bifulco, Spence, et al., 2019).

This chapter will explore the use of technology in psychological measurement and treatment. We will then look at CLEAR in more detail – how it was developed, what it consists of and how it can be used. The chapter will outline the benefits of CLEAR such as data handling, use of pre-programmed algorithms for complex variables, the ability to add different questionnaires to tailor to different studies and the personal feedback provided upon completion. This is followed by the limitations of the measure including its reliance on self-report, its relative ability to mimic an interview and the skill required of the respondent to objectively rate their own emotion-laden events. We then look at the psychometric properties of CLEAR which has been tested on a student and middle-aged sample. Finally, we explore the potential further development of CLEAR and its research and clinical applications going forward.

Advancing technology in measurement

Over the past couple of decades, psychological research, assessment and treat-ment have experimented with new technology. Indeed, research studies, inter-ventions, journals and books abound on the subject (Luiselli & Fischer, 2016; McKenna, Joinson, Reips, & Postmes, 2007). Online application is particularly suited to questionnaire or checklist methodology, and there are various secure platforms which host these. Early 21st-century discourse has been interested in how online surveys mimic traditional paper and pencil applications. In the *American Psychologist*, Gosling and colleagues debunked six negative preconcep-tions surrounding the internet (Gosling, Vazire, Srivastava, & John, 2004). They found that samples from the internet were generally more diverse than tradi-tional samples, participants were motivated and that results were consistent with more traditional methods. Studies have also found that digital survey methods are comparable to face-to-face questionnaires in terms of reliability and validity (e.g. Buchanan, 2007; Gosling et al., 2004; Hiskey & Troop, 2002; Weigold, Wei-gold, & Russell, 2013). So, two issues are pertinent to this approach – whether samples are collected via the internet and the issue of the measures themselves being posted online.

Psychology research on the web is not only limited to survey methods but is also used for varied psychological testing (Buchanan, Johnson, & Goldberg, 2005; Chuah, Drasgow, & Roberts, 2006). Furthermore, web-based experiments are also shown to produce similar results to laboratory-based studies. A study compared several experiments done in the lab with web-based equivalents on their own online testing environment (TestMyBrain.org) and found that despite the fact that participants are self-selected, unsupervised and uncompensated for their time, the data showed comparable results to the lab environment (Germine et al., 2012). Other studies have researched the recruitment of participants through web-based platforms such as Amazon's Mechanical Turk (MTurk):

> Amazon Mechanical Turk (MTurk) is a crowdsourcing marketplace that makes it easier for individuals and businesses to outsource their processes and jobs to a distributed workforce who can perform these tasks virtually. This could include anything from conducting simple data validation and research to more subjective tasks like survey participation, content modera-tion, and more. (https://www.mturk.com/)

Here, participants are paid for their participation and tend to be from a more diverse group than other internet samples. In addition, data acquired from studies using MTurk have been shown to be as reliable as those from the more traditional data collection methods (Buhrmester, Kwang, & Gosling, 2016). A study by Ramsey and colleagues looked at whether being in a lab compared to being web-based made a difference to participants following instructions (Ramsey, Thompson, McKenzie, & Rosenbaum, 2016). They found that all participants performed similarly whether in the lab or online and that if anything the MTurk sample was more likely than the students to read instructions properly (op cit).

We are aware of one other online approach to measuring life events, but this is broader and examines key experiences over the life course including childhood. The Stress and Adversity Inventory (STRAIN) has recently been published showing good reliability at re-test and good overlap with the Childhood Trauma Questionnaire (Slavich & Shields, 2018). However, it has not been validated against an equivalent interview – such as the ALPHI (Bifulco, Bernazzani, Moran, & Ball, 2000) adult adversity interview or indeed the CECA (Bifulco & Moran, 1998) childhood interview. It enquires about 55 different stressors – including 26 acute life events and 29 chronic difficulties – over the lifetime. In homage to LEDS, it follows up self-report responses with further probing questions. However, these are limited given time for completion is only 18 minutes. It does not aspire to replace the 12-month LEDS measure of life events and difficulties. Thus, our own approach using the CLEAR, we believe to be the only one attempting to replicate this interview online – attempting the 'third generation' of contextual life events approaches.

We are aware of the numerous benefits of using the web for data collection, many of which impact directly on research cost and thus overcome practical interview limitations. First, all data inputted by the user can be downloaded directly into files ready for statistical analysis taking the laborious task of data entry out of the equation. Second, given the potential to reach a much wider range of people, it gives researchers the opportunity to capture more heterogeneous samples and those geographically spread and cuts down considerably on costs as recruitment time is much quicker. Anonymity can also play a big factor in recruitment as the data is sent straight to a server anonymously rather than being passed back to a researcher; participants can choose to withdraw at any point without the pressure of the researcher being present. There are, however, pitfalls to the approach, including the online design aspects of the tool and how this may influence the user's responses and engagement. Issues include how many questions should be on each screen or how being invited to take part in a survey can impact on the user. However, in terms of web formatting, research shows that for survey methods, format does not influence the quality of data collected (Gosling et al., 2004). Therefore, usability will probably not affect the reliability of the data collected. The larger issue is the quality of the self-reported information given.

CLEAR – an online assessment of life events

CLEAR was fashioned in line with the LEDS interview with adaptations to make it more applicable for online use. The look of the online tool was designed with a modern feel, with different colours used as a border and a white, clean finish with small icons to represent different domains and with a friendly and readable format. (The images shown here in figures are monochrome for publication reasons.) We also took into consideration the sensitive nature of the research and the tone of the information that was being collected – it needed to be serious but also friendly and accessible. CLEAR was also designed to be compatible for use on multiple devises (e.g. laptop, iPad) and using various web browsers.

The underlying programme was designed by YouthinMind[1] as already utilised in the roll out of the Strengths and Difficulties questionnaire (Goodman, Ford, Simmons, Gatward, & Meltzer, 2000) online to schools and clinics. It thus followed the same structure in terms of collating information by respondent, including on a prospective basis, in a secure and anonymised system. The CLEAR layout involves several steps to guide the underlying structure. Once online consent has been obtained, the user is directed to the front-landing page which enables them to start filling out their demographic characteristics. This includes date of birth, ethnicity or living with a partner and children. Additional demographic questions appear in the relevant domain sections, such as the work section including type of job, management responsibilities, number of hours of work and so on. Other questionnaires are also added to the site and accessed in 'More about you' (see Figure 6.1). In our project, this included the General Health Questionnaire[2]; the Warwick-Edinburgh Mental Wellbeing Scale[3]; an itemised physical health checklist and the Vulnerable Attachment style Questionnaire (Bifulco, Mahon, Kwon, Moran, & Jacobs, 2003).

In LEDS, life events are split into ten different domains. CLEAR has differentiated 'Children' from other relationships creating an additional domain.

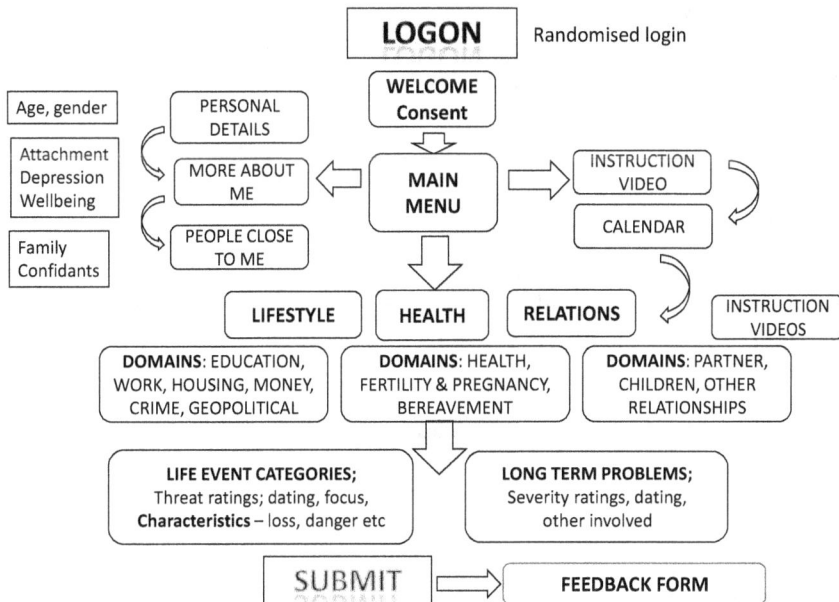

Figure 6.1 Map of CLEAR elements.

CLEAR follows the same LEDS concepts but arranges it into a computer-friendly format with an initial three arenas (Lifestyle, Health and Relationships) so that the user is not overwhelmed with the hundred or more potential event categories when first seeing the task. The Lifestyle arena subsumes the categories in education, work, housing, money, crime and geopolitical for both life events and difficulties/long-term problems (see Figures 6.1 and 6.2). The overall Health domain includes events and difficulties in health, fertility and pregnancy and bereavement categories. The Relationships category encompasses life events and difficulties in marital/partner, children and 'other' relationships (family of origin and confidants) categories. For each domain, a list of possible event categories are presented to the user as a reminder of what events might have occurred over the past year for the user to check if present. If they have experienced a life event, then this directs them to menus which are dependent on previous respondent choices to further categorise and rate the event on different characteristics. The link with any long-term problems can be made through a menu that presents any entered on to CLEAR by the user. Long-term problems are queried early on in the menu, and these can be returned to at any point to refresh or add to. Each life event identification then repeats the same process, with a large number of event categories potentially covered, but with most individuals only endorsing a few subsets and not having to negatively score the remainder. The full CLEAR takes around 45–60 minutes to complete, and a shortened one is under development to take a planned 40 minutes. All responses are automatically saved as the respondent progresses, and it can be completed over multiple sittings at the user's convenience. Below, we provide an example of how an event is recorded on CLEAR. All the prompts asked in the process are to help the user refine the event in order for them to be able to give a more precise rating at the end. Here is an example taken from the CLEAR project showing some of the screen shorts and an event concerning 'Health'.

Example – CLEAR health event

The event selected concerned a car accident that the female respondent experienced, her partner being with her in the car. The car was badly damaged and she suffered from concussion; her partner was unhurt. This involved a visit to hospital where she was kept in overnight, but later released and told to take bed rest and to move as little as possible. An X-ray showed that there was no lasting damage. She was off work for three weeks. Figure 6.2 shows a basic screen with the initial 'health' option. Figures 6.3–6.4 show further ratings.

In Figures 6.3 and 6.4, the respondent describes the health implications of a car accident that happened in May of that year to her and her partner. It can be seen that she rated 'accident' which affected mainly her; that it '*involved a degree of significant shock*' and '*involved injury*'. She did not tick that the event led to long-term illness or disability, or that she was off work for several weeks, or that there were financial consequences since these did not apply in her particular case.

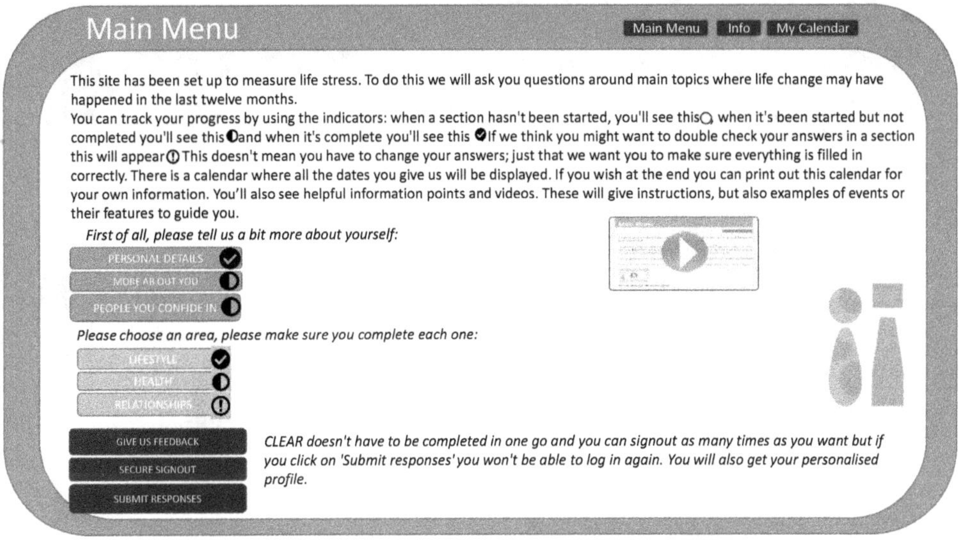

Figure 6.2 Initial CLEAR Health option.

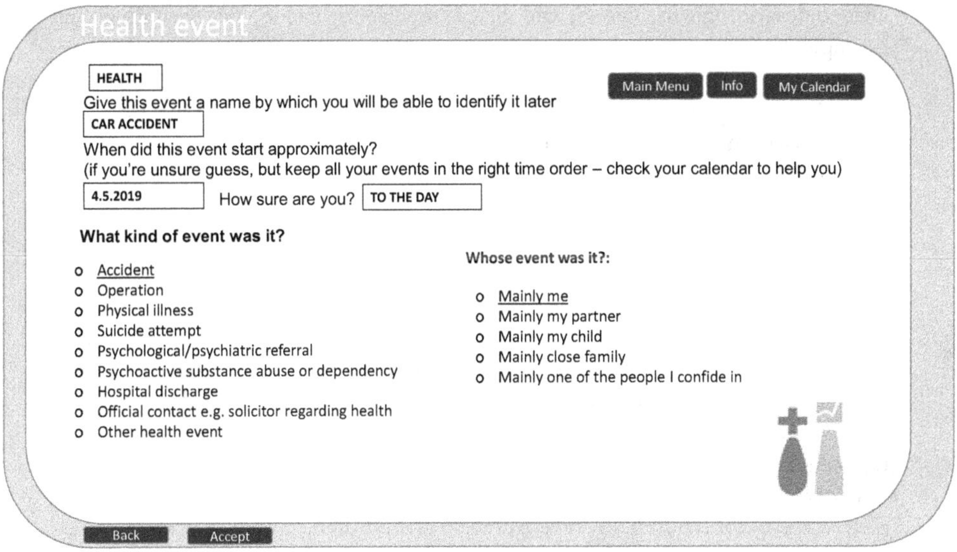

Figure 6.3 Options on health event menu – more event descriptors.

The respondent then rates the description of the event and how she felt. Then, further characteristics about the event, including her qualitative description, were collected. Two videos are accessible at this point in the system for participants to watch in order to receive guidance about how to rate severity.

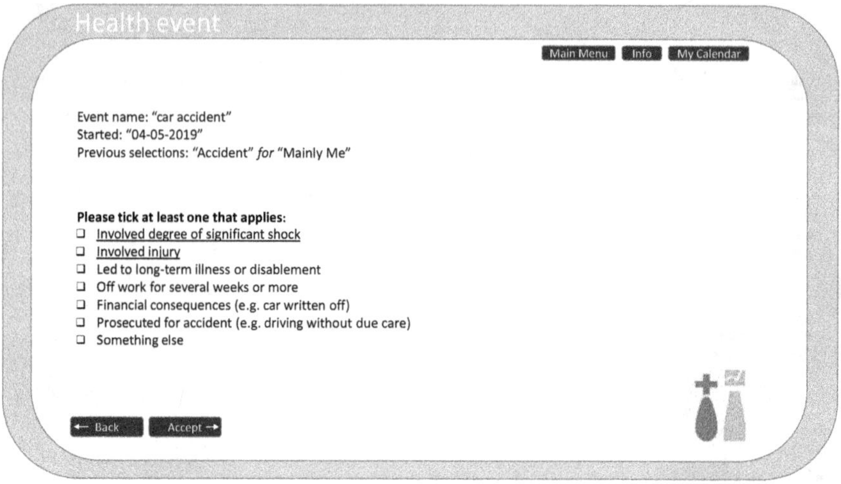

Figure 6.4 Further specification of event.

Finally, the respondent is asked to rate the event both in terms of its *threat* (how negative the event was) and how *positive* it was. Instructions are given in terms of a video describing what *threat* is and then a more specific video per domain giving examples for each level of threat. The videos use simple animation with voice-overs as these are considered applicable to all ages and are emotionally neutral. This also avoids the possibility of respondents over or under identifying with scenarios based on superficial characteristics of actors (such as age, race or gender). Respondents are then asked to rate for *short-term threat* (in the first day or two) and *long-term threat* (10–14 days later).

Life event 'Threat/unpleasantness' is rated on a five-point scale.[4] Ratings 1–3 are classified as a 'severe' event (this includes the LEDS upper (a) and lower (b) moderate ratings) and 4–5 are non-severe events. Each has a descriptor which implies the level reflected – 1: Extremely damaging to lifestyle, relationships, goals and security; 2: Very damaging to lifestyle, relationships, goals and security; 3: Moderately damaging to lifestyle, relationships, goals and security; 4: Somewhat damaging to lifestyle, relationships, goals and security; and 5: Little/no damage to lifestyle, relationships, goals and security.

In this example, the respondent rates *2: Very damaging to lifestyle, relationships, goals or security* for the first few days (short term) and then rates *3: Moderately damaging to lifestyle, relationships, goals, security*. This reflects a higher level of threat at the time of the accident when the health outcome was unclear, but somewhat lower threat once it was clear that her concussion was expected to get better, although it left her bed bound and off work for some weeks. This was then counted as a severe event. The respondent also rates it affected '*both me and someone else*' and that '*no long-term problem was related to the event*'.

The scoring of a LEDS *severe event* is calculated in CLEAR using a pre-coded algorithm enabling the rating to be carried out automatically applying the

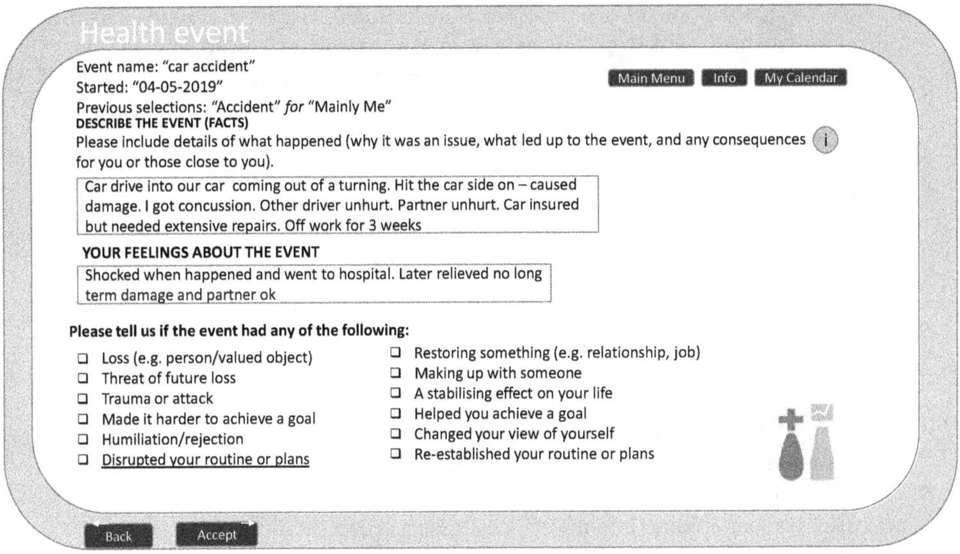

Health event

Event name: "car accident"
Started: "04-05-2019"
Previous selections: "Accident" *for* "Mainly Me"
DESCRIBE THE EVENT (FACTS)
Please include details of what happened (why it was an issue, what led up to the event, and any consequences (i)
for you or those close to you).

Car drive into our car coming out of a turning. Hit the car side on – caused
damage. I got concussion. Other driver unhurt. Partner unhurt. Car insured
but needed extensive repairs. Off work for 3 weeks

YOUR FEELINGS ABOUT THE EVENT

Shocked when happened and went to hospital. Later relieved no long
term damage and partner ok

Please tell us if the event had any of the following:

- Loss (e.g. person/valued object)
- Threat of future loss
- Trauma or attack
- Made it harder to achieve a goal
- Humiliation/rejection
- Disrupted your routine or plans

- Restoring something (e.g. relationship, job)
- Making up with someone
- A stabilising effect on your life
- Helped you achieve a goal
- Changed your view of yourself
- Re-established your routine or plans

Main Menu | Info | My Calendar

Back | Accept

Figure 6.5 Rating aspects of event.

following criteria that make an event severe: (i) 1 marked, 2 high-moderate on *long-term contextual threat (higher)* or 3 *lower-moderate* and (ii) is 'self' or 'joint'(respondent and someone else close) focused. When an event is only focused on someone other than the respondent, it does not meet criteria for a *severe* event. In the example above, whilst both respondent and her partner were involved, the health implications were only for her – so it qualified as 'self-focused'. Figure 6.5 shows additional ratings including felt response.

Security of the CLEAR system

It should be stressed that the CLEAR system is very different from an online questionnaire such as reproduced in qualtrics. It has a more elaborated architecture which can identify an individual (through randomised password) and utilise this for any follow-up investigation to link records. It can be personalised for any individual new project. Given that CLEAR is an online application, web-based security is a key concern of the electronic architecture. All participants only enter data under an ID number and personalised password, and therefore no names/contact details are entered onto the CLEAR system. Two security devices were incorporated. The CLEAR servers are built from CentOS Linux which is a secure variant of Linux; this has no services or ports installed, except what is strictly necessary for CLEAR. A firewall was installed to further restrict access to the server. Normal operating system conventions are followed with regard to passwords and user accounts (i.e. long enough passwords with mixed case letters and numbers, only known accounts are installed). All data are stored on the MySQL database which has its own security mechanisms and added proprietary security mechanisms. All access to data is through trusted client tools through accounts specifically enabled for remote access and/or through programs. Finally, all applications to the CLEAR architecture may be themselves password-protected and accessed via an encrypted communications channel. Maintenance of confidentiality and ensuring that those entitled to access the system do not create insecurities once the data or reports are outside the system are carefully monitored.

CLEAR findings

Whilst the CLEAR application was online, the sample investigated was carefully selected (offline) to be suitable for answering the research questions around severe life events and depression. Given only an online questionnaire of symptoms was to be used, it was deemed necessary to select a previously identified clinical depression group and matched controls to enable comparisons for clinical disorder risk (see study 11, Appendix 1). The questionnaire symptom scale (GHQ) is only a proxy measure of depression. However, additional questions were added to the GHQ for the dating of initial and peak symptoms to approximate to onset. It was also deemed appropriate to select a student group recruited from a London university which increased the age range studied and the ethnic diversity.

The Depression Case Control Sample (DeCC) was originally a UK multi-centre, case–control sample selected for a study of unipolar depression in midlife white respondents (Korszun et al., 2004). These depressed patients were originally identified through psychiatric clinics, hospitals, general medical practitioner surgeries and media advertisements and had experienced at least two episodes of unipolar depression. Matched controls were recruited through general medical practices across the UK and were excluded if they had a personal or first-degree relative with a history of psychiatric disorder (Korszun et al., 2004). Permissions were given to recontact this sample after a ten-year period for the CLEAR study. It comprised 202 adults (mean age 57.6; range 36–75 years), of whom 75 were recurrent depression cases and 127 controls. There were more females overall and due to the prior genetic sampling constraints for ethnicity, all were White. Most of the DeCC sample had partners and children and were educated to at least a degree level. There were 126 students (mean age 21) over half of which were partnered, but few had children. This was a more diverse sample with 37% from Black Asian and Minority Ethnic (BAME) groups.

The depression results reported here utilise only the DeCC groups for purposes of sample homogeneity with regard to age and selection (Bifulco, Kagan, et al., 2019). The student sample is also used in the reliability and validity findings as well as in the next chapter examining positive events. In order to establish whether CLEAR-rated events can predict depression in a similar manner to LEDS – both a group analysis (prior clinical vs control) and a combined group analysis (to examine life events characteristics and attachment vulnerability to GHQ depression) were utilised. The group findings are shown in Table 6.1. Results revealed that depression was differentiated as expected – with 33% of the sample having GHQ depression in the prior clinical group versus 10% in the

Table 6.1 Group comparison CLEAR odds ratio of rates in clinical group versus control. DeCC sample (n = 202)

Clear ratings	OR (clinical vs control)	Confidence interval	p Value (from χ^2)
GHQ 12-month depression	9.48	4.29–20.98	p < 0.001
Severe event (higher 1–2 threat)	6.20	2.78–13.84	p < 0.001
Severe event (lower 1–3 threat)	2.35	1.31–4.27	p = 0.005
Non-relationship event	2.46	1.35–4.46	p = 0.003
Relationship event	1.59	0.61–4.12	p = 0.332 (ns)
Loss event	2.88	1.39–5.93	p = 0.003
Danger event	2.71	1.29–5.70	p = 0.007
Humiliation event	5.40	2.24–13.04	p < 0.001
Goal frustration event	1.19	0.55–2.57	p = 0.655
Trauma event	10.74	2.31–49.93	p < 0.001
Attachment insecurity	4.43	2.38–8.23	p < 0.001
Anxious attachment style	2.80	1.54–5.07	p < 0.001
Avoidant attachment style	6.70	3.56–12.82	p < 0.001

Table 6.2 Rates of depression by event type and attachment style – CLEAR study (DeCC sample groups combined n = 202)

Risk factor	OR for depression	Confidence interval	p < (from χ^2)
Severe life event (lower threat)	3.59	1.70–7.30	<0.001
Severe life event (higher threat)	6.72	3.00–15.00	<0.001
Loss severe event	3.78	1.70–8.10	<0.001
Danger severe event	4.81	2.10–10.68	<0.001
Humiliation severe event	6.38	2.70–15.09	<0.001
Goal frustration severe event	2.95	1.28–6.74,	<0.01
Trauma severe event	5.83	1.75–19.44	<0.005
Attachment insecurity	4.68	2.27–9.65	<0.001
Anxious attachment style	2.59	1.24–4.99	0.008
Avoidant attachment style	2.69	1.34–5.41	0.004

control group. The prior clinical group also had higher prevalence of severe life events and features of severe events such as loss, danger, trauma and attachment vulnerability (see Table 6.1). The figures in the table show the odds ratio for the risk factor or depression in the clinical group versus the control group. Thus, GHQ depression showed that the clinical group had a 9.8 higher risk of disorder in the study period than the control group and severe event 6.20 higher. Thus, CLEAR was able to differentiate these groups in the expected manner. Only relationship severe events were not differentiated by group.

When severe events were then examined in relation to depression in the combined group of clinical and control respondents, significant odds ratios were found for risk factors and depression (see Table 6.2). Thus, the presence of a severe event was associated with 3.5 times the rate of depression using a lower threat cut-off (1–3 on the five-point scale) but rose to 6.72 times with a higher cut off (1–2 on five-point scale). The characteristics of severe events also raised risk of depression – the highest being humiliation (6.38 increased rate of depression) and trauma event (OR = 5.83). Loss was somewhat higher than danger (4.81 and 3.78, respectively) and goal frustration only 2.78.

When insecurity of attachment style was examined as a vulnerability, having an insecure style was associated with depression (OR 4.68) and this held for both anxious style (OR 2.59) and avoidant style (OR 2.69).

Finally, the contribution of both severe life events and insecure attachment style was examined in predicting depression. Each contributed independently (severe event; OR 3.68, Wald 7.88, 1df, $p < 0.005$) and (insecure attachment style 2.64, Wald 5.42, 1df, $p < 0.02$). An interaction was evident, but just short of 5% significance level (insecure attachment * severe event: OR 7.37, Wald 3.75, $p < 0.053$). Therefore, CLEAR seemed to be able to replicate the main LEDS findings from earlier studies described in Chapters 2 and 3 and thus indicate predictive validity. Both severe life event and attachment vulnerability contributing to the depression model and the interaction term was only marginally short of statistical significance.

When this analysis was repeated utilising only the severe event prior to the estimated onset as determined by GHQ dating of symptoms, the same model held.

The checklist life events measure LTE-Q had been incorporated into the CLEAR site as an additional measure of life events for the purpose of comparison with CLEAR. This allowed respondents to score whether a severe event in a particular category had occurred. When the checklist LTE-Q events were similarly examined to GHQ depression, no significant relationships were found. The presence of any one LTE-Q severe life event did not relate to depression: 27% versus 26% (OR 1.06, $p = 0.90$). However, there was a modest association between LTE-Q overall score (with all checked events summed) and General Health Questionnaire symptom score ($r = 0.19$; $p < 0.001$). When the LTE-Q events were grouped by category for presence or absence and examined in relation to depression, none were significant (Health OR 1.39, $p = 0.29$; Work OR 1.35, $p = 0.29$; Crime OR 1.26, $p = 0.40$; Fertility OR 1.62, $p = 0.09$; Housing OR 1.42, $p = 0.17$).

Thus, even when respondents are scoring checklists within the same online CLEAR system, they are not associated with depression. Therefore, it can be seen that CLEAR was a much more effective predictor of depression than the checklist LTE-Q with which it was administered.

CLEAR reliability

The CLEAR project incorporated a test of reliability (test–retest) for 60 respondents, 20 from each of the three groups. They repeated CLEAR at first contact and then again around a month later. Analysis was undertaken using intraclass correlations (ICCs). CLEAR showed very good reliability for demographic ratings (average 0.92, range 0.79–1) on 14 scales including age, gender, ethnicity, partner status, work, children, pregnancy history and parents alive. This also held for the overall number of events (0.89) and number of severe life events recorded at both time points (85.4%, ICC = 0.60, $p < 0.001$). There was good association (using ICC) for category of event (0.91), focus (0.64) and long-term threat (0.63). There were 94 long-term problems reported by this subsample, with only 36% of participants reporting no long-term problem at either time point. The agreement for severe long-term problems was however, only modest (0.38, p < 0.001). Yet category agreement was high (0.97) with persons involved (0.65) and peak severity (0.62) moderately associated.

When the reliability of the LTE-Q was examined across the two test points, this was less good at ICC = 0.57. This rose slightly for those events 'active now' to 0.67.

CLEAR validity

Validity was tested by comparing CLEAR responses to ratings from a parallel face-to-face LEDS interview with 30 participants (10 from each group). These were balanced; so half completed the CLEAR first and the other half were interviewed first. When the comparison of demographic variables across the two methods was examined, there was good agreement. For example, using ICCs, these ranged from 0.74 to 1.00 for 20 variables involving age, ethnicity, education, work, children and housing.

When life events were compared, it was immediately evident that LEDS generated many more life events than CLEAR. Thus, of 184 life events across both measures, 94% (167) were identified by LEDS but only 36% (67) by CLEAR – although most of these latter overlapped with LEDS (75%). When long-term problems (difficulties) were examined, a similar picture emerged where the interview identified 78% (73) and CLEAR 38% (36).

Before considering why fewer events and long-term problems were picked up by CLEAR, investigation of the overlap of the event characteristics for those in both measures was first examined to look at reporting agreement for event characteristics. Here, there was good agreement. Thus, for short classification of event, the ICC showed 0.74 and focus 0.83 with threat 0.89. This meant that severe event identification was relatively good (0.67). The following general findings became evident in explaining some of the lack of agreement however: first, the midlife group consistently achieved higher agreement than the student group and obtained higher overlap of the two methods overall. This maybe because the students rushed completing the measure due to time constraints or lack of commitment. Or it could have been because their lives proved more complicated and unstable with more life events occurring and therefore more complex aspects of events to consider than the settled midlife group. The second more general factor showed that events focused on the individual scored as having higher agreement than those focused on close others. This suggests that respondents are more focused on their own events and show more consistency in reporting those. The next section will examine why the CLEAR system recorded fewer life events than the interview with case examples.

Reasons for missing events in CLEAR

A small qualitative analysis of the interview narratives and the brief descriptions of events on CLEAR allowed for an exploration of why many events were not identified in the CLEAR system. Both sets of events with descriptions were collated by respondent and examined for various elements:

- **Clustering of events:** The LEDS identifies experience at each point of its occurrence – for example, diagnosis of an illness, tests taken, hospital admission or operation. Instances were found whereby the overall problem situation was identified in both systems but with fewer events in the cluster identified in CLEAR. Therefore, knowing whether the 'severe' events were identified in CLEAR becomes important for provoking agent analyses.

- **Event/Long-Term Problem misclassification:** LEDS has characteristic ways of categorising events based on what are considered to be the most salient characteristics which in contrast can vary in the CLEAR system. For example, a row with an alcoholic husband who was drunk would be rated under 'partner row' but could also be considered in respondent report as a 'husband health issue'. Similarly, the LEDS differentiates between acute and chronic experience, whereas long-term experience may have been incorrectly included as a single life event in CLEAR rather than a long-term problem.

- **Rogue responders:** In at least one case, the respondent entered no events whatsoever on CLEAR, but in the LEDS interview had a total of 13. The researcher analysing commented: '*His pattern of completion of CLEAR is a little odd. He's completed the personal details and the other questionnaires. However, he didn't enter details for any people he is close to. He didn't enter anything (not even demographics) for the Health domain (including Health, Fertility, Bereavement). He did though complete the Lifestyle and Relationships domains, but for each individual area he indicated that he had no events or LTPs. He had ticked the box to say that he'd completed the site overall*'.

- **Student unstable lifestyle:** The student group had nearly double the number of events of the midlife groups in LEDS. Some had high rates of change in their lifestyles; for example, frequent changes in friendships, partnerships, accommodation and part-time jobs. This factor may have created recall or identification problems of the various happenings, with only a few reaching threshold for self-report inclusion.

- **Reasons for discrepancies in the categorisation of long-term problems:** Classifications were sometimes problematic on CLEAR, for example, 'husband's alcoholism' could be rated in either health or relationship domains; similarly, 'daughter depletes savings due to health issues' could be rated as money or health. The 'other involved' categorisation could also be unreliable depending on misidentification of the focus of difficulty (i.e. who was the actor) versus its resulting impact on others. For example, events involving the respondent's health were sometimes rated for their impact on partner.

These findings provide insight into the respective benefits of the two methods of data collection and how the two systems vary. It also suggests ways in which CLEAR can be improved to enable more valid scoring. CLEAR shows good test–retest reliability and good predictive value, but its comparison with the LEDS itself reveals a weakness in specifying categorisation of the *same* events. However, when singular events were rated in the two systems, they were good at providing similar ratings, including severity level.

The following case examples illustrate some of these similarities and differences in how events and long-term problems are rated across the two systems.

Case examples of CLEAR – LEDS comparison

Evie – clinical group

This 74-year-old married woman was retired and living with her husband. She has three grown-up children who live away from home. Her events include her husband's and son's health. In addition, she has events concerning her brother-in-law's illness and death. Whilst in-laws would not routinely count as 'close others' for events, in this situation, Evie and her husband were very involved as they frequently visited the brother-in-law who lived abroad during his terminal illness. They had to make various funeral arrangements when he died. However, neither of them was emotionally close nor had a confiding relationship. The death of a friend was also reported but she was not a close confidant – again this not usually counted in the LEDS scheme.

Evie completed CLEAR before having her LEDS interview, and the following list of events indicates when they were captured by either or both methods. She had no depression in the study period (see Figures 6.6 and 6.7).

LTE-Q score: When this was examined, Evie had a score of three events – family illness, death of family member and death of close friend. None of these were severe on either LEDS or CLEAR.

This LEDS interview shows some good overlap with CLEAR in the rating of both events and long-term difficulties. One of the scoring issues is over the status of non-immediate family events (e.g. brother-in-law) and non-confidant friends. Usually, both are excluded as events in the LEDS, unless the respondent has an unusual amount of involvement. In this interview, the brother-in-law was included (but not rated as severe since it had no lasting implications for Evie); the second – no close friendship – was not. The former did require unusual involvement, and the latter did not. In contrast, neither was self-reported as severe on CLEAR. This also influences the long-term problems which are scored on CLEAR, but not included on LEDS.

One instance where CLEAR did not match well with LEDS classifications was on the husband's heart disease diagnoses and forecast of operation (proceeding the operation). On LEDS, the diagnosis and forecast was rated as an event, but on CLEAR, Evie rated the diagnosis and operation together with the latter associated severity – which was low due to a positive outcome. However, the outcome of the operation was not known at the earlier point, so a severe life event due to the uncertainty of the situation and associated risk of danger was missed by CLEAR. Despite this differentiation, both measures gave the difficulty a marked rating for the period when husband was at risk.

Which measure	Description of event
Identified event	
Interview alone	**Husband's heart diagnosis**: husband diagnosed with a serious heart problem and told operation was needed **(Severe event LEDS)**
Both methods	**Husband's heart operation**: it was successful and with good prognosis **(Non-severe – both methods)**
Both methods	**Brother-in-law's hospitalisation** for terminal cancer whilst living in Spain **(Non-severe – both methods)**
Both methods	**Brother-in-law dies (Non-severe – both methods)**
Interview alone	**Son's knee problem**: adult son has a chronic knee problem and is told he will need an operation **(Non-severe LEDS)**
Interview alone	**Son thyroid diagnosis**: treated with medication **(Non-severe LEDS)**
Both methods	**Friend dies**: friend from years ago dies from cancer - not close confidant **(Incident/not event - LEDS; Non-severe CLEAR)**

Figure 6.6 Analysis of Evie's events by CLEAR and LEDS.

BOTH	**Arthritis/Heart:** has arthritis and ongoing mild heart problem for the last 3 years. She goes once a year to the consultant and it hasn't got any worse as the medication she takes keeps it under control. Side effects make ankles swell so also has to take water tablets. Causes some breathlessness and slows her down. **(Non-marked LEDS; Marked - CLEAR)**
BOTH	**Husband's heart condition (Marked – both methods)**
BOTH	**Brother-in-law terminal cancer hospitalisation and death (Marked – both methods).**
CLEAR alone	**Next door leak/new meter:** the leak affected the electrics in Evie's house. Had to buy new metal boxes and wires. Couldn't use the washing machine for some time – wires for appliances were all over the kitchen. Had to have a new electricity meter installed and they were over-charged £300, and the company would not return it. Involved constant phone calls, but eventually was sent the money. **(Marked - CLEAR)**

Figure 6.7 Evie's long-term problems/difficulties by methods used.

Frank – clinical group

Frank is a 50-year-old white British man, divorced and living alone. He has one adult child. His profession is as a musician, but he is now registered blind and unable to work. He has other health problems and money difficulties.

He was interviewed first with LEDS and then completed CLEAR. It can be seen that many of his events described below were only identified by interview, but there was better overlap with long-term problems/difficulties. Frank had a depression during the year – the dating of peak suggests that this was after his job rejection (see Figures 6.8 and 6.9).

On the LTE-Q, Frank ticked illness, unemployment and burglary as having occurred.

In this example, it can be seen that Frank had more events and difficulties scored by LEDS. However, the events missed by CLEAR were all non-severe, with the only severe event occurring being scored as such by both methods. For long-term problems, the eyesight problem was rated as marked by both methods, but the additional work difficulty only rated by LEDS – presumably CLEAR had subsumed it with the health problem. However, both systems agreed on the money difficulty rating.

Thus, it can be seen by examining particular cases that reasons for discrepant ratings are at times understandable in terms of the inclusion or exclusion criteria and the collapsing of events or events and long-term problems in their reporting.

LEDS ALONE	**Accident walking in Lake District**: nearly fatal but results in only cuts & bruises (Non-severe LEDS)
BOTH METHODS	**Job rejection for academic post**: perceived as last chance to get work and enhance his career. The job would have been possible to undertake with his disability **(Severe event; Loss; goal frustration – both methods)**
LEDS ALONE	**Funding rejection for a grant application (Non-severe LEDS)**
LEDS ALONE	**Identity theft/emails hacked**: there was police involvement, but no loss of money **(Non-severe LEDS)**
LEDS ALONE	**Broken microphone**: required £1000 for replacement **(Non-severe LEDS)**
LEDS ALONE	**Unpaid fellowship application successful**: with access to expensive resources **(Non-severe-positive LEDS)**
LEDS ALONE	**His musical composition work accepted at prestigious academy** (Non-severe-positive LEDS)
BOTH METHODS	Arthritic pain: High level of pain **(Severe event on CLEAR and LEDS difficulty)**

Figure 6.8 Frank's life events in both methods.

BOTH	**Health: eyesight** failing through macular degeneration; registered blind, impacts not only on daily life but on his career as an artist. **Marked** – both methods)
LEDS	**Health: osteoarthritis** with mild chronic pain and uses steroid medication **(Not marked LEDS - CLEAR identified as event)**
LEDS	**Identity theft**: mail stolen, no money taken but receiving requests **(Not marked LEDS)**
LEDS	**Work**: as a sculptor his work is affected due to health. Has failed with gaining grant and job applications **(Marked – LEDS)**
BOTH	**Health: lung & bowel problems** causes breathlessness and digestive issues **(Not marked – both methods).**
BOTH	**Money difficulty:** Due to ill health and not working 'my expenditure exceeds income. I cannot access some benefits due to having savings.' Has to make sacrifices and live more frugally **(Marked - both methods).**

Figure 6.9 Frank's long-term problems/difficulties in both methods.

This needs to be examined in the further development of the CLEAR to ensure greater consistency of reporting. However, the online approach provides a very promising new avenue of measurement.

Advantages of CLEAR

Less social desirability bias

One well-documented advantage of such an online approach is that respondents are more likely to report honestly due to the anonymity of web-based measures compared to speaking to an interviewer (Musiat, Hoffmann, & Schmidt, 2012). One study compared social desirability distortion on computerised interviews to face-to-face interviews (Richman, Kiesler, Weisband, & Drasgow, 1999) and found that when revealing sensitive information such as drug use or risky behaviours, respondents were more likely to reveal information on the computerised equivalent which they believe is due to the privacy, anonymity and the ability to go back and change responses. Interviewing for life events can often bring up embarrassing or sensitive topics, and having an online system may help people to think about their events in a more open manner. Additionally, CLEAR enables the respondent to go back into the system and change any prior responses after reflection, which may encourage more thoughtful response.

Less resource-intensive and more detailed

The rationale for developing the CLEAR system as aforementioned was to attempt to capitalise on the benefits and pitfalls of questionnaire and interview approaches. Web-based measures/interventions, in general, and CLEAR, in particular, are less resource-intensive given that the respondent completes their rating in their own time and data is directly inputted and coded. Given this lower resource-intensive method of gaining information, what benefits does it have over a traditional life events check list? It has similarities to the question-naire in that it is self-report but improves on this first through the capture of much more detailed information and gives instruction at each step on how to make the judgements required. Thus, it includes within each category an extensive number of different life events that may have occurred – based on the vast experience of the LEDS interview. It allows for multiple completion of a category, for example deaths of more than one specified close other. This contrasts with the LTE-Q where the respondent is asked 'have any of your im-mediate family died?' or 'have any of your other close relative or close friends died?' allowing only one positive response to each. CLEAR enables the user to fill out a life event for each time someone dies and determines detailed in-formation such as the relationship, the prior closeness and, importantly, the timing of the event. Those identified as close contacts (family of origin, partner and children and close confidants) are all identified at the start of the task by name/nickname. In addition, fields are provided for qualitative description of events and responses.

Captures timing and sequencing of events

Being able to date life events is extremely important in marking a causal rela-tionship with onset of disorder (Hunt, Bruce-Jones, & Silverstone, 1992; Monroe, Slavich, Torres, & Gotlib, 2007). Whilst this is easily achieved in interview, it is rarely achieved in questionnaires, indicating that sequence and time lag cannot be ascertained. CLEAR requires event dating and provides a calendar to aid with this. The date certainty is queried (e.g. 'to the day', within one to three days, three to five days, within two to three weeks, month, etc.). Finally, all events are placed in a personalised calendar which the user can refer to as they go along as a visual reference and is updated as life events and anchoring events are added (e.g. holidays, birthdays).

Creates CLEAR personalisation and feedback form

CLEAR is personalised throughout the system in a variety of ways which have been found to enhance user experience (Dijkstra, 2005). First, the respondent identifies those who are close to them by first name, and this populates the meas-ure and personalises menu options. Utilising names enhances engagement in on-line measures by heightening attention to information given (Lyketsos, Nestadt, Cwi, & Heithoff, 1994). The CLEAR personalised calendar is continuously up-dated with the respondents reported life events which they can, on an ongoing basis, check for accuracy and timing. Additionally, on completion of CLEAR, the user is given a personalised feedback report based on the information that was inputted. This feedback can be tailored to the study or for clinical purposes.

This is common practice in certain websites (e.g. TestMyBrain.org) in exchange for participation in experiments and is seen to encourage participation (Germine et al., 2012).

Allows addition of related questionnaires

Another benefit of using CLEAR is that multiple questionnaires can be added to the system depending on the study variables or for added clinical use. These questionnaires are part of the opening page which has a section called 'More about you' and once added can be programmed to give scores for individual items plus composite variables. In our study, we added measures investigating attachment style, wellbeing and depression. The personalised feedback included a summary of this information along with their individual life events and long-term problems. This feedback can also be adapted as an interface which can be sent to clinicians to aid practice.

Disadvantages of CLEAR

Lower event capture

Although CLEAR may be more time efficient than an interview, it does not capture the same degree of information and accuracy, even though it performs better than the LET-Q checklist (Bifulco, Spence, et al., 2019). The system which is designed to mimic the interview process has not been and is unlikely to ever be able to capture the information gathered by a trained interviewer who can use individualised probing questions until satisfied the information is complete. In a similar vein, although we attempted to 'train people on the job' in how to rate *threat*, whether this can be done to the same degree of accuracy as the interview is questionable given the length of time it takes to train individuals in the LEDS rating system. Furthermore, whether it is indeed possible to take the subjective element out of their perceptions of experience and rate it in a manner that is comparable to the aims of the LEDS needs further study.

Recall accuracy unknown

One of the great disadvantages with retrospective measures, for both checklist and interview, is memory recall (Uher & McGuffin, 2010). Interviews can help with this in some ways as the interviewer prompts the participant, but questionnaires and other self-report cannot rely on this. When designing and piloting CLEAR, we took this into account and looked for methods to enhance self-report in the measure. One method was through the use of the calendar which can aid in a more accurate reporting of events (Drasch & Matthes, 2013) even going back a number of years (Belli, Shay, & Stafford, 2001). Adding in further personal dates such as birthdays and anniversaries can boost recall (Lyketsos et al., 1994). In addition, allowing users to complete the system over a number of sessions allows them to change or edit their responses and gives them more time to think through their responses which has also been shown to be important in aiding recall (Belli et al., 2001). Furthermore, it reduces respondent fatigue as the user can stop and start as they wish; something that they would not be able to do in an interview.

Loss of personal expert approach

One of the advantages of interviewing as a means of collecting information is the dynamic between investigator and respondent. A rapport can be built whereby trust develops in the interaction, and the interviewer can seek out consistency and detail in the account produced. A sensitive interviewer can see if a respondent seems to be holding back, if their account is confused or muddled and whether they seem to be downplaying the seriousness of events described. This can help in utilising probing questions for further information to elicit a better narrative overall. Such inconsistency in reporting tends to be related to vulnerability, in particular to attachment style (Main, Kaplan, & Cassidy, 1985).

One consideration of how best to use the CLEAR versus the LEDS maybe around population (representative samples) versus vulnerable samples. The idea of utilising both approaches in mixed methods may be feasible. The current state of play is that CLEAR is in the process of being shortened with more non-optional menus provided to further guide respondents. Some unnecessary demographics are also being reduced. At this point, a second validity exercise will be under-taken with a representative group to establish the sites comparison with LEDS further. However, there are other options for the use of CLEAR meanwhile – one is to utilise a face-to-face interview but use the smart online system for researcher rating – this swiftly processes the information automatically into usable data and also provides a feedback report.

Future uses of CLEAR for research purposes

We can speculate here on future uses for CLEAR and ways it may be used as en-tirely online respondent-only, or a guided online approach with the interviewer, or for some populations as an interview with an easy online rating system for the investigator to complete later. The team are now in the process of finalising a shortened version of CLEAR-2, and a new validity analysis will be undertaken on a representative group.

Epidemiological research

We see CLEAR as having most use in population-based study where large sample sizes across a wide geographic area are studied prospectively. For ex-ample, to further investigate disparities in health through investigating severe life events and long-term problems on a prospective basis. This could also be utilised to check for mental health and morale on a wider scale, for example, with nationwide issues such as pandemics or political issues such as asylum seeking after war conflict or even looking at events in times of economic depression or austerity. This perhaps has something in common with the Mass Observation study during the Second World War (Wing, 2007), which is now being extended for the Covid-19 pandemic.[5] The ease and low cost of use would facilitate this approach. This would entail the online use of CLEAR, although a robust mixed-method approach would utilise more intensive face-to-face investigation of a selected subgroup.

Research – genetics

As discussed in earlier chapters, 'G × E' studies of depression have utilised life event approaches along with micro-genetic investigation, some using interview and other checklist approaches. Usually, such studies require large numbers of respondents. Many research groups have spent considerable time and effort investigating the relationships of genetics and environmental stimuli, such as life events, especially in the area of depression (Monroe & Reid, 2008; Uher, 2008) and bipolar disorder (Hosang et al., 2010). Some teams have found the sought interaction, whereas others have not (Fisher et al., 2012; Risch et al., 2009), and the choice of life event tool has been implicated with interviews faring better (Uher & McGuffin, 2008). Although CLEAR does not appear to pick up events as thoroughly as interview, it certainly improves on checklist questionnaires, and its validity may indeed be increased by its use in mixed-method designs.

Students in higher education

CLEAR is currently being used in a student population to look at life events and emotional disorder as well as grade achievement over the course of undergraduate study. We know that rates of emotional disorder are high in student populations as well as experience of negative life change. Universities are committed to aid in improving student experience and the conditions for positive learning. In addition, student mental health has over the past number of years been both highlighted in the popular media and has received considerable attention in both the academic (Macaskill & Denovan, 2013) and policy (Health, Health, Excellence, Society, & Psychiatrists, 2011) spheres due to the high rates of mental health issues within student populations (Ibrahim, Kelly, Adams, & Glazebrook, 2013; Wynaden et al., 2014). Mental health and wellbeing is often highlighted, but the actual effects of life events themselves are not widely recognised and being able to assess student life events and then provide appropriate support may mitigate the effects of life events for more vulnerable individuals. In addition, we also know that interpersonal events can put individuals at risk for developing depression, particularly so in students (Hysenbegasi, Hass, & Rowland, 2005; Reyes-Rodríguez, Rivera-Medina, Cámara-Fuentes, Suárez-Torres, & Bernal, 2013), where the university years can be a period of flux for relationships due to new social opportunities and students moving away. We are currently in our third year of looking at CLEAR data from students to help us understand in what ways life events impact this particular population with respect to their mental health, wellbeing and academic achievement (Spence, Rodriguez-Bailey, et al., in press). Using technological measures to assess stress levels can help university support services and potentially aid study progression along with success on a wider scale.

Analysis of the student findings using CLEAR indicates that severe life events and a lack of social support are both associated with depression. Additionally, depression and poor social support are associated with lower academic achievement in first-year exams with a three-way interaction between severe life events, depression and social support (Spence, Rodriguez-Bailey, et al., in press). Ongoing investigation is looking at this group prospectively to investigate whether this holds across years of study and to final degree categorisation. Harnessing such methods could be a significant aid for university staff in helping student achievement and increasing wellbeing.

Health service-users

In the health sphere, technological approaches to life event assessment can aid identifying risk in perinatal services, in diabetes clinics and cardiovascular services where stress is a major contributor to health outcomes (Alloy, Abramson, Safford, & Gibb, 2006; Brown & Harris, 1989; Craig & Brown, 1994; Mooy, De Vries, Grootenhuis, Bouter, & Heine, 2000). Having a detailed understanding of a patient's psychological profile, in terms of their recent severe life events and other vulnerability or lifestyle measures, might aid in providing a more holistic approach to the medical perspective of lifestyle risk. Thinking of how individuals manage chronic health conditions in what might be difficult personal circumstances may lead to better patient-treatment adherence. This is already established in terms of difficult interpersonal attachment styles (Ciechanowski, Katon, & Russo, 2005). Trying to manage a chronic health issues is known to be difficult in and of itself and some clinics (e.g. diabetic, cardiovascular) offer psychological treatment to help the client understand their barriers to self-care regarding their conditions. Perhaps, in addition, utilising a methodology such as CLEAR may help both health and psychology clinicians think about the sociological and psychological consequences of life events and the impact it has on service users. A pilot project started in Derry, Northern Ireland with the Health Trust for Perinatal services showed that the CLEAR measure could be adapted for women registered with antenatal services to establish both life events and vulnerability during pregnancy in relation to postnatal depression outcomes. This initial work showed feasibility of using the CLEAR in this context.

Clinical implications – technology in psychological treatment

Online methodology has not limited itself to psychology research, and its use also extends to therapy and to clinical diagnosis. In terms of the latter, there is an online method which was created from the same approach as the CLEAR by Robert Goodman and his team for both symptom scales (SDQ) (Goodman, 1999) and clinical interview (DAWBA) with children and adolescents, which is now extended to adults (Goodman, Ford, Richards, Gatward, 2000). The Difficulties and Welbeing Assessment covers a number of psychiatric diagnoses and can integrate self-report and assessments by others including practitioners. It is a package of interviews, questionnaires and rating techniques which can generate clinical diagnoses on children, adolescents of adults. It is now developed by Youthinmind for rolling out not only to schools but also to young adults.[6] There is of course great potential in linking this to the CLEAR site for additional clinical assessment online.

Psychological treatments on the internet, particularly for cognitive behavioural therapy (CBT), abound. These have become particularly important during Covid19 social distancing regulations. A recent systematic review of online CBT identified 2,078 studies as a starting point for their meta-analysis comparing face-to-face CBT to therapist-guided internet ICBT (Carlbring, Andersson, Cuijpers, Riper, & Hedman-Lagerlöf, 2018). Similarly, Andersson and colleagues report that there are around 300 controlled studies of online interventions (Andersson, Titov, Dear, Rozental, & Carlbring, 2019). As accessing face-to-face psychological therapy can be difficult due to limited supply, online applications are viewed as a way of improving access for many more individuals as they can be delivered remotely with minimal expense (Andersson, Topooco, Havik, & Nordgreen, 2016). ICBT is available for multiple disorders such as depression, social anxiety, panic disorder and post-natal depression.

Research has shown promising results for ICBT with some studies finding web-based treatment that include clinician contact to be as effective as face-to-face therapy (Carlbring et al., 2018) and yet other studies finding ICBT to be slightly superior (Andersson, Rozental, Shafran, & Carlbring, 2018). There is also a debate as to whether having some therapist contact, for example, email support or initial face-to-face contact is important for the treatment process. Differing levels of therapist contact are typically offered, ranging from none, to assessment before starting treatment, to contact throughout. Results tend to show that therapist-guided ICBT is superior to non-guided. In addition, guided ICBT compares favourably to traditional face-to-face therapy for different disorders (see Andersson et al. (2019) for a comprehensive review). There have also been reports of the long-term benefits of online psychological treatment approaches (Andersson et al., 2018). In an 18-month follow-up of ICBT, Knaevelsrud and colleagues found that improvements were sustained for symptoms of PTSD, depression and anxiety. Similarly, sustained effects for ICBT for a range of clinical disorders were also found (Andersson et al., 2018).

Online treatment applications are not just limited to ICBT. In a recent meta-analysis for online Acceptance and Commitment Therapy (ACT) (Hayes, Strosahl, & Wilson, 1999), 59 studies were identified and 10 met criteria for inclusion in the study. Results showed web-based ACT to be effective for depression although not for anxiety and general wellbeing (Brown, Glendenning, Hoon, & John, 2016). The authors note the importance of web-based therapy tools in the context of overall public policy, where responsibility is being shifted from the service provider to the individual to help themselves in terms of lifestyle and health decisions. Psychodynamic therapy (PDT) has also been tested online. A study compared a ten-week psychodynamic-based online treatment in a randomised control trial versus a support intervention for participants diagnosed with depression (Johansson et al., 2012). They found that internet PDT was superior to the control condition. Other therapies which have been adapted online are mindfulness, interpersonal psychotherapy and solution-focused therapy-based programmes (Andersson et al., 2019). Additionally, treatments have been expanded to smartphone apps enabling them to reach more users for a number of different conditions (Chandrashekar, 2018).

A separate advantage to the expansion in the availability of online treatments is that it facilitates research with randomised control trials to take place more easily. Internet psychotherapy research is less demanding on resources due to ease of data collection, less researcher time needed and other resources such as therapy room availability (Andersson et al., 2019).

Thus, there have been great advancements into the digital field for research and clinical practice. The facility of online applications to reach out to wider audiences and still maintain high-quality research or clinical outcomes is hugely important as it combines both convenience with a method which has an accumulating evidence base. However, when it comes to measuring social risk factors, there has been limited application. Most typically, online systems upload questionnaires onto secure sites and download the results. These are online checklists open to the same limitations as their paper and pencil versions. Clearly, there is a need for a sophisticated technological system capable of assessing life events that could take advantage of the benefits of online measurement, the rigours and theoretical basis of interview measures and move on from the many limitation of checklists. On the backdrop of this need, a new method was born – the CLEAR – a comprehensive, usable, theoretically relevant measurement of life events combined with the advantages of online sophistication.

Use of CLEAR for psychological services

CLEAR could easily have a role in clinical services, including those conducted online. CLEAR is client-led, involves little clinician time, could aid assessment and provide details of life events and their ratings to aid accurate formulation about the lead up to psychological disorder. Although this is usually done in an assessment session, there is not the time to dedicate a whole session on life events and difficulties, so having the online input could give the clinician valuable information as a background to sessions. Reported events could be discussed in the following sessions to check no context has been overlooked. This could also be an opportunity for discussing the importance of characteristics such as danger, loss and humiliation and relating these to vulnerability. Verbal feedback received about CLEAR from research participants in our study indicated that some people found the actual experience of completing CLEAR to be therapeutic in and of itself, as the user was able to have an understanding and a visual representation in the calendar of what had occurred over the past year. One user commented that completing CLEAR helped them to see how much they had been through and how well they had actually dealt with it. The feedback provided can serve to tease out the real extent of many events and could consequently encourage more realistic estimations of coping or endurance.

A clinical area where CLEAR might be most suited is for low-intensity therapy or manualised online CBT (Ruwaard, Lange, Schrieken, Dolan, & Emmelkamp, 2012). Here, formal assessment of the clients' life events and difficulties are not routinely undertaken, only symptom assessment for treatment suitability (Helgadóttir, Menzies, Onslow, Packman, & O'Brian, 2009). CLEAR could provide the role of identifying precipitating factors required for CBT and potentially also vulnerability estimates. Thus, CLEAR could be useful for Improving Access to Psychological Therapy (IAPT) services. As discussed in the final chapter, these have been developed as a model in the UK for individuals with mild to moderate anxiety or depression, created for those who would not meet criteria for direct clinical work but could benefit from help from mental health teams (Layard, 2006). In 2017, IAPT services were seeing around 960,000 people a year with around 60% receiving evidence-based treatment (Clark, 2018). This approach is based on a stepped care model where individuals can be offered time-limited therapy based on assessment according to NICE 2004[7] guidelines (Kendall, Pilling, Whittington, Pettinari, & Burbeck, 2005). Low-intensity therapy is manualised treatment and is often given by a Psychological Practitioner who does not have a clinical qualification but bespoke training for low-intensity work. One of the criticisms of low-intensity therapy is that the interventions are only minimally tailored for the client due to the lack of in-depth training experienced by the worker and the manualised treatment approach. CLEAR might be a method of helping both the client and practitioner to have a better understanding of the clients' problems and life context. Either before an initial session or during the first one, the client could be shown how to complete CLEAR in their own time or with support. Following completion of CLEAR, the client and clinician can both receive the personalised feedback for further discussion.

Discussion

Whilst internet research, with clinical and psycho-educational application, has abounded over the past two years in the field of psychology, life events research methodology has not kept up with this trend. CLEAR is one of the first of this new generation of tools to look at life events and difficulties in a format which is easy to use, engaging and can capture a wide range of experiences. We suggest that this platform will lead to some new thinking around how life events can be captured economically and how this could revivify its research application and give aid to clinical practice.

There are caveats – this first iteration of CLEAR does not capture all relevant events, but those it does capture, particularly those severe, tend to be rated accurately and in detail. A new version of CLEAR is in development which is shorter (some demographic detail omitted) but also more directive (respondents asked to check all possible events in a domain rather than simply the one selected). This is likely to increase event capture. However, some ingenuity may be required in getting the best fit of online tools in combination with face-to-face measures. For example, large population surveys, where only a proportion of respondents are vulnerable, may give sufficient accuracy for a sole online approach. However, for vulnerable samples and those clinical, it may be that face-to-face questioning may helpfully supplement CLEAR in some way. This could involve joint use of the online system and a face-to-face interview, using the online tool for rating, or subsequent checks on events that may have been missing when explored verbally. Further research will be needed to check the utility of such approaches and the extent to which they add to predictive models.

Although not without its disadvantages, we see CLEAR as a new way forward to help capture the intricacies of life events which have interested researchers and clinicians alike for many decades. We hope it will inspire researchers, clinicians and policy makers to think more about how technology can aid in both capturing and understanding the complexities of our ongoing life stories.

Notes

1 https://youthinmind.com/
2 http://www.psicothema.com/pdf/3564.pdf
3 https://warwick.ac.uk/fac/sci/med/research/platform/wemwbs
4 The LEDS utilised a 4-point scale but then differentiated 2a high moderate and 2b low moderate. CLEAR has created a 5-point scale. In line with LEDS 1–3 on, this new scale is utilised for severe event category, although some analyses have also utilised 1–2 termed high severity.
5 http://www.massobs.org.uk
6 https://youthinmind.com
7 https://www.nice.org.uk/media/default/about/what-we-do/into-practice/measuring-uptake/niceimpact-mental-health.pdf

Section 3

Positive life events, recovery and wellbeing

7   Positive events and recovery

As described in earlier chapters, life events research has tended to focus on negative experience in relation to emotional disorder, particularly depression. However, life changes can be positive, and fewer studies have focused on the impact of positive life events on reduction of depression or increase in wellbeing. This is in part because most life event checklist scales only include negative events. Yet recovery from depression can be attributed to experiencing positive events and the reduction of difficulties. If these were understood more widely, it could usefully influence intervention and treatment. Positive events are as varied as negative ones and include aspects such as promotion at work, starting a new partner relationship, giving birth or receiving financial gain. Research indicates that these types of event can have positive impacts on mental health (Headey, 2006). They can increase feelings of subjective wellbeing and life satisfaction, and we will outline how they are associated with recovery from depression and anxiety (Brown, Lemyre, & Bifulco, 1992). In this chapter, the positive characteristics of events will be outlined as will their role in aiding recovery from disorder using the Bedford Square team research. In addition, in this chapter, the role of positive self-esteem as a 'robustness' factor for resilience will be examined in increasing the impact of positive events. In examining positive factors, we will also examine the role of crisis support and good coping at the time of a severe event in relation to averting depression. Finally, interventions linked to coping and support with life events will be outlined.

Different dimensions of positive life events

In the LEDS interview, a positive event is one that is capable of arousing a strong positive emotion. Thus, it would be expected to confer gratification, enjoyment or satisfaction and also add meaning to life and to felt security. This would include events that bring about positive change by reducing the severity of difficulties or social deprivation (e.g. an overcrowding housing difficulty ended by moving to a larger property) or positively creating a new role (e.g. becoming a parent). In relation to the ASIA model described earlier, positive events can increase security (e.g. success in getting a promotion and better pay), fill a needed attachment role (e.g. finding a close confiding friend) or help the individual realise a goal for achievement (e.g. passing an important exam) or increase identity (e.g. citizenship being granted). These events may also improve the quality and consistency of existing relationships when difficulties diminish (e.g. reconciliation with sister following period of not speaking). Therefore, some events can be positive in their own right (e.g. passing an exam, winning a large cash prize), whereas others are positive because of a change from prior negative conditions (e.g. achievement despite prior failure; new relationship after a period of isolation).

As with other events, positive events have first to merit event status by denoting sufficient life change (i.e. indicate public, behavioural or environmental change) as opposed to a change of mind or intention or feeling. Rating of positivity is only made *after* the event is already identified and when any positive implications are apparent. It is possible for an event to have both positive and negative implications (e.g. a divorce finalised; parent's recovery from a stroke resulting in some disability). As with negative events, all of the various categories of event described earlier (e.g. education, housing, crime, partner) can involve positivity. In the LEDS, positivity is rated on a four-point scale with only the top two points ('marked' and 'moderate') on long-term outcomes qualifying it as a discrete 'positive event'. In this next section, we focus on the underpinning research undertaken with the LEDS and positive events. This to provide a key to understanding what makes a life event positive and how this can impact on the individual.

Socio-environment and positive events

Whilst negative life events are significantly related to social deprivation, the converse does not appear to hold for positive events, that is, they are not increased by affluence and privilege. Also, objective life circumstances appear to explain little of the variance in personal happiness levels (Lyubomirsky & Ross, 1999; Lyubomirsky & Tucker, 1998). This seems to be for two reasons. First, because some positive events mark the ending of a long-term problem, the latter having been linked to social adversity. So, the positivity is relative to prior deprivation. Second, individuals with positive social environments (e.g. wealth or status) do not seem to reap as much positive emotion from positive events. Thus, a study shows that wealthier individuals showed less 'savouring' ability to enhance and prolong positive emotional experience (Quoidbach, Dunn, Petrides, & Mikolajczak, 2010). The interpretation given is that with the increase of social expectation, less enjoyment is experienced with small pleasures in life. This is also known as the 'experience stretching hypothesis' – that experiencing the best things in life spoils people's enjoyment of lesser pleasures (Gilbert, 2006). It would appear that positive events are therefore evenly distributed by class and groups, but differentially appreciated.

Testing positive events and recovery

Research by members of the Bedford Square team, utilising the LEDS in community research, identified key dimensions of positive life events in relation to recovery from clinical depression and anxiety. These included two sets of characteristics: those positive events involving anchoring/stabilising and those fresh start/enhancing events (see Figure 7.1 for definitions). Those anchoring/ stabilising all occurred after a period of deprivation or adversity, often indicated by a LEDS difficulty of an unstable situation. They thus equate with feelings of relief and renewed hope when life challenges and difficulties begin to abate, end or are followed by a new positive trajectory towards greater security. These represent different stages in such alleviation of burden – for example, 'relief' when a difficulty first looks to be reduced, 'routinisation' when a situation becomes more predictable and finally 'anchoring' when there is solid evidence of a stable positive future. These align with an increase in stability of roles, relationships, finances, housing and other domains. These events have been mostly linked with anxiety reduction. Enhancing/fresh start events involve situations when a new positive element occurs in a person's life as a source of reward or pleasure. Thus, a new relationship or role or possession. This can at times occur after a period of deprivation or difficulty and occur in stages such as 'de-logjamming/blockage removal', 'potential fresh start' with indication of the desired positive event more likely and finally 'fresh start' when the new opportunity actually arises. These events have been mostly linked with depression reduction and are summarised in Figure 7.1.

These events were first examined using the LEDS in the early 1990s in the Islington study (see study 3, Appendix 1), with a focus on those with recovery from clinical levels of either anxiety or depression or mixed conditions (Brown et al., 1992). The analysis aimed to see if particular types of positive events preceded each type of recovery. Only those individuals with an episode of clinical depression or anxiety which had lasted at least 20 weeks, and where there was a recovery or improvement to subclinical or 'no disorder' levels were included in this analysis. This comprised 92 women with anxiety disorder and 67 with depression, and the analysis compared events in phases during the disorder episode and those prior to recovery in the same women, thus using different phases occurring in the same women's lives as comparison points. Results are shown in Figure 7.2 and indicate that significantly more of those with fresh start type of events had recovery/improvement of depression (odds ratio 9.87). In addition, significantly more phases with an anchoring type event preceded a recovery/ improvement of anxiety (OR 5.75) and mixed events related to recovery from mixed disorder. Thus, the relationship of specific types of positive life events to recovery/improvement points was confirmed.

Positive evaluation of self

In Chapter 4, negative evaluation of self (NES) was shown to be a vulnerability factor for new onset of depression. The detailed interview measure utilised by the Bedford Square team also had parallel positive scales including positive attributed-self and positive role-competence – these two scales were combined for analysis into a positive evaluation of self (PES) index. As with the negative

---

Stabilising events – linked to anxiety recovery

Anchoring event – a likely increase in security following increased regularity/predictability in an activity or relationship. This included finalising divorce or separation, confirming a partner relationship (cohabitation or marriage), more settled housing (e.g. change from renting to ownership), more secure employment (unemployed to regular work). Also included were less finalised events such as:

- o Routinisation – individual returning to previous activities (resuming work after maternity leave)
- o relief – event likely to help resolve a problem for someone close to the individual e.g. partner getting a job after being unemployed.

    relief→routinisation→ anchoring (least to most stabilising)

- •

    Enhancing events – linked to depression recovery

Fresh start event – change in a situation which gives hope following a prolonged difficulty or deprivation. The individual is always the focus of the event. An example would be a single mother with limited finances and unable to find work, finally getting a job. It also includes reconciliation after estrangement of six months or more with someone close or rehousing after a period of housing difficulty due to overcrowding. Also included were less finalised events such as:

- o Potential fresh start – when the situation is not yet resolved – e.g. offer of rehousing after difficulty overcrowding, but new house not yet available.
- o De-logjamming/blockage removal – event clears the way for a future solution but substantial difficulty still present. For example, agreeing to leave a job after period of harassment, but without having a new job to go to.

Blockage removal → potential fresh start → frest start (least to most enhancing)

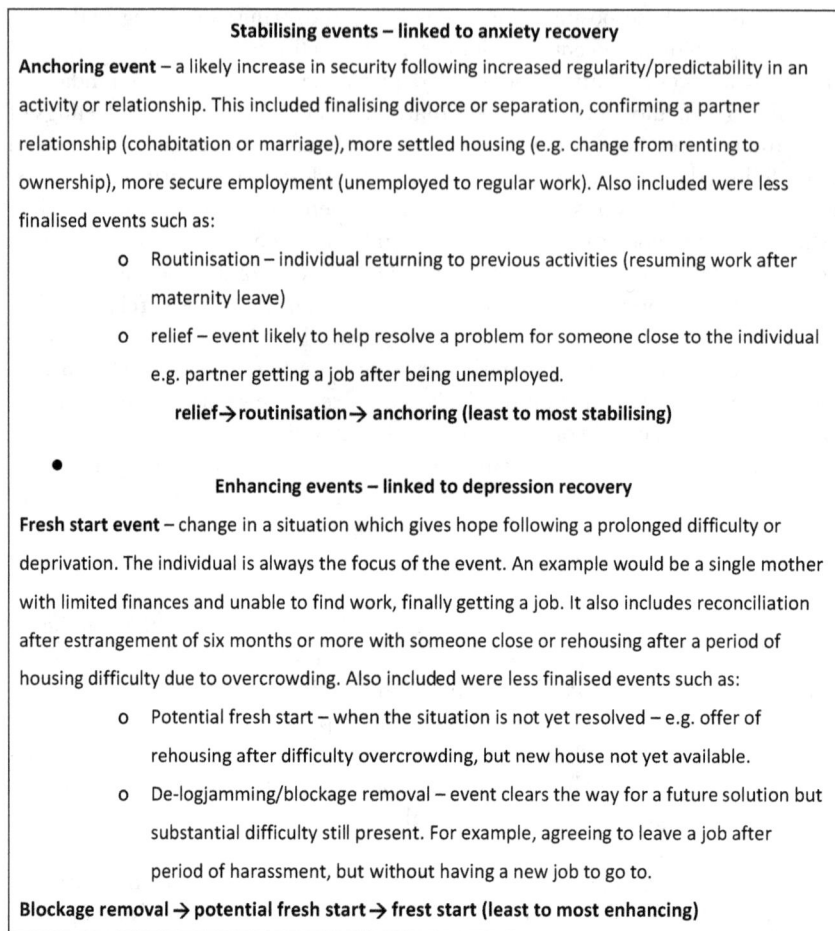

Figure 7.1 Features of LEDS-positive events in recovery.

scales, the SESS interview (O'Connor & Brown, 1984) utilised scoring of interview comments on a range of items involving PES-attributions (e.g. perceptions of intelligence or attractiveness) and role performance (e.g. perceived competence as a parent or as a support figure to a friend). Global self-acceptance, or rather its lack, was only included in the negative NES index. However, for the dichotomised index, a 'marked' rating was required on at least one of the scales, since moderate levels of positive estimation were rather commonly held. As well as scoring highly on the negative (NES) or positive (PES) index, an individual could score highly on both scales to reflect different roles or attributes in a more complex self-estimation, or indeed on neither perhaps indicating a weak sense of self overall. It was considered important not to average these negative and positive

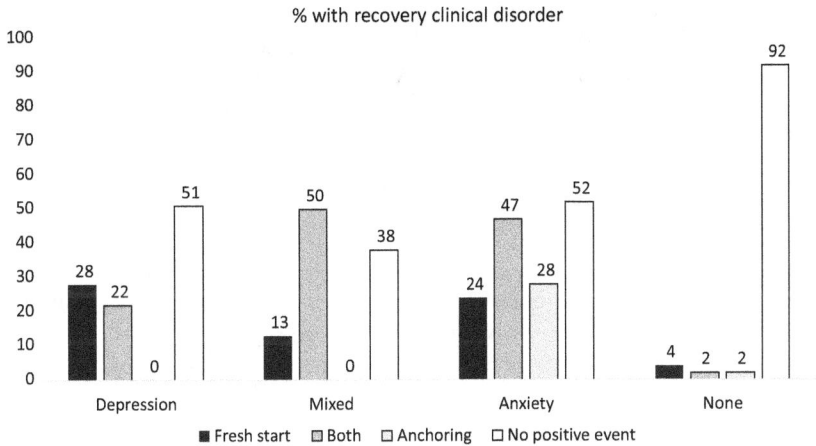

Figure 7.2 Positive events and recovery from clinical disorder.

items but rather to reflect peaks of ratings on both ends of the spectrum. In other words, seeing one's self as high on intelligence would count towards PES, but low on attractiveness would feed into NES. Having no opinion of one's attributes would feed into low ratings on either index. The self-esteem findings are summarised below, and all involve the Islington representative sample (see study 3, Appendix 1) (Brown, Bifulco, & Andrews, 1990b).

Examples of positive self esteem

This woman described her view of her personal attributes in response to the different questions asked:

> 'I'm usually the same, day in, day out, morning, noon and night - pretty cheerful, I do think that's a good way to be! I do feel confident – but not overconfident – but enough to get what I want. I like to think I'm easy to get on with, and easygoing, which I am. I can be sympathetic and then again I can be hard when its needed.' (She sees both as positive). 'I can be efficient if I put my mind to it and I do get things done' I tend to give way to other people. I'm all for the easy way out if that keeps the peace.' (She sees this as positive as well). 'I think I'm pretty easy - affectionate, about right'. She tends to say what she thinks. When asked about her intelligence, she said 'Average'. She says she's 'not particularly attractive, but it never bothers me'. 'I'm not quiet. I'm not boisterous either. I'm just in between really'. 'I'm very happy with the way I am'.

Another woman described her positive evaluation of her roles. She was a single mother, divorced and lived with her children and does not go out to work but is a homemaker. She stated that she is *'very* good' as a mother. She's also *'very* good' as a housewife and 'couldn't imagine not being a housewife'. About her divorced status, she said with some pride: 'I am very independent since I've been divorced'. Also, 'I'm a very sympathetic friend… a very trustworthy friend, and valued by my friends. They find me easy to get on with'. She says that she 'copes well as a single parent'.

Correlates of PES and depression

Utilising a continuous PES score (summing the full four point ratings on both scales), correlations were found with a range of scales involving relationships and roles (Brown, Bifulco, Veiel, Andrews, 1990). Those significant included positive quality of interaction across relationships (i.e. warm, enjoyable, stimulating and humorous times together) and in roles (with partner, children and work), lack of social isolation and positive security regarding housework. For single mothers, correlated scales also included social participation, social and financial resource availability.

When positive aspects of self-esteem were examined, PES was found to be protective of depression among women *with* severe life events – 19% of those with PES had an onset of depression compared with 32% without (Brown, Andrews, Bifulco, & Veiel, 1990). However, these effects were reduced when there was a let down of expected social support at the time of the severe event (see later in the chapter for further discussion). Figure 7.3 shows the beneficial effect of PES on onset but only when expected social support was present (i.e. left-hand columns particularly the first) (Brown, Bifulco, & Andrews, 1990a).

PES was also examined prospectively in relation to recovery of chronic episodes of depression and found to predict recovery or improvement (among 40 respondents all (100%) with prior PES recovered and 50% of those without)

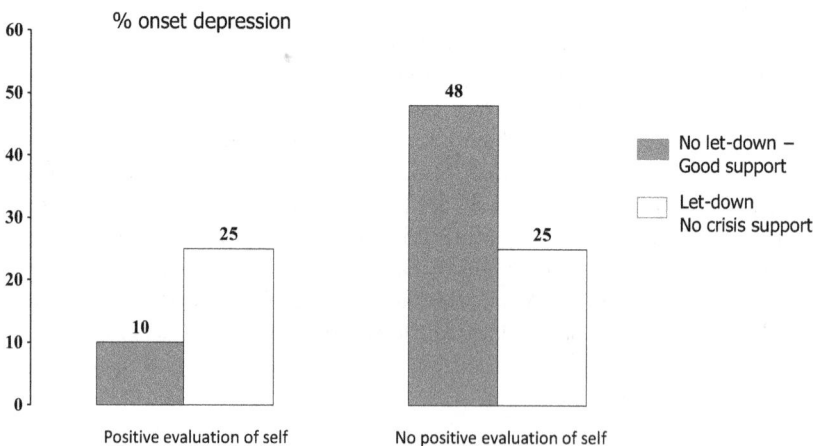

Figure 7.3 PES, crisis support and onset of depression.

(Brown et al., 1990b). There was also an effect of a fresh start event, with both independently required to predict recovery from depression (op cit).

PES was also a contributor to depression recovery. In addition, PES and the absence of NES related to a greater frequency of positive events (particularly fresh start and difficulty reducing). PES added to the impact of such positive events in predicting recovery/improvement. There was also a small suggestion that the prior presence of such positive self-esteem was related to the initiation of positive events by the individual (Brown et al., 1990b). Thus, taking initiative in finding a job, having a disabled son return home from residential care and even getting pregnant whilst living in overcrowded social housing to force rehousing seemed to be related to PES-related actions (op cit).

Example of depression recovery

Lucy had been depressed for two years initially precipitated by problem neighbours and poor housing, and her symptoms maintained by deterioration in the relationship with her partner, who had also become depressed, and behaviour problems in her son. Lucy had a part-time job which she was able to sustain. Her comments about herself were both negative and positive. In terms of PES, she made a number of positive comments:

> I've got a lot of will power; I'm not stupid, I'm very intelligent; I'm very good at English and things; I'm attractive; I can make up my own mind about things; I'm a good mother. I feel proud that I keep a nice flat... I can cook meals; I'm good with old people, I always put people first.

During the follow-up period, Lucy's marriage started to improve, her husband spent less time out in the evenings, spent more time with her and the children, for example, taking them out at weekends. He also offered more emotional support. They made a decision to have a second child, Lucy became pregnant and a healthy child was born. They then became eligible for new social housing since they needed another bedroom. This was arranged and Lucy and her family moved house, going to a better area and getting away from the difficult neighbours. Her depression reduced to subclinical levels. [PES at first contact. Positive events – (i) birth of baby; (ii) moving house. These were fresh start events.]

Coping and crisis support – averting depression

A further issue relevant to positive outcomes for those suffering from severe events is the issue of coping, including crisis support. These are the immediate responses to the events as they unfold, requiring speedy coping responses and alert support from close others. Thus action to avert a depression rather than actions to aid recovery. However, these can be relevant to the interventions to be discussed later in the chapter and so will briefly be outlined here, as emerging from the Bedford Square team projects.

Whilst the time lag between a provoking event and onset of emotional disorder can be relatively brief, there is still opportunity for crisis coping and the potential for accessing crisis support in the immediate aftermath. A number of informal (i.e. non-practitioner) interventions have been based around the confiding/emotional support axis. This includes befriending interventions (described below) as well as self-help groups where people with similar types of crisis offer each other support. It is also central to the psychotherapy interaction where the client confides their thoughts and feelings in relation to crises and is able to accept meaningful support and guidance.

One of the key elements around crisis support is the importance of full confiding. This is the key element of accessing support. It is not a simple construct. It involves telling another trusted and close person at the time of the crisis the events that have caused concern and upset. It involves disclosing feelings as well as circumstances. The act of confiding helps the individual process the event psychologically (those who deny elements of an event typically do not confide). Positive emotional support from the other is required for effective 'social support' which can help to 'soothe' or regulate emotions, shows care and acceptance and can provide help and advice.

Successful confiding represents a number of features. First, it requires the individual to be able to communicate need when under stress; and second, it assumes the presence of a close and trusted figure with prior history of supportiveness to whom the individual can turn to. Third, for resilient support, it also requires alternative sources of confiding support should the first choice be unavailable. Although, both bad luck and timing may also be involved – more than one support figure may be lost in a crisis (e.g. mother's untimely death makes both her support unavailable and that of a grieving sister, both circumstances outside the individual's control). Timing concerns whether support figures are available in what may prove to be a window of only a few weeks to offer crucial support before depression takes hold.

The representative Islington prospective study (study 3, Appendix 1) undertaken by the Bedford Square team demonstrated that confiding was central to both coping and crisis support at the time of a severe life event. The Coping Schedule provided additional interview questions utilised alongside the LEDS (Bifulco & Brown, 1996). This queried about subjective coping response to severe events and related difficulties or 'crisis' complex. A crisis complex, for example, could include a partner difficulty linked to a sequence of severe events involving partner separation. Coping questions would thus focus on the whole situation, not only on single events within it. Scales reflecting practical coping response (seeking knowledge about the crisis, practical actions taken), emotional response to the crisis (distress, anger), attributions for the crisis (blame, self-blame) and cognitive avoidance (downplaying, cognitive avoidance or inferred denial) were all utilised (Bifulco & Brown, 1996). This also included crisis support questions which asked whether any of the individual's previously identified close support figures were contacted and provided emotional support at the time of the crisis (Brown, Andrews, Harris, Adler, & Bridge, 1986).

Findings showed that one positive cognitive factor, that of downplaying/ looking on the bright side, was protective of disorder. Thus, none of the 18 vulnerable individuals who experienced a severe life event and responded with high downplaying became depressed. This reflected individual ability to control negative emotions around the crisis and use social comparison to make the situation seem comparatively better than it may be for others, thus feeling lucky or grateful. Other findings showed an increased risk of depression from those who used negative coping strategies including self-blame, pessimism or inferred denial of the problem (Bifulco & Brown, 1996). These can be seen to further link to the negative cognitive triad described by Beck to enact or heighten vulnerability.

Examples of good coping – downplaying

An example is of a woman who gave birth to a baby with Down's syndrome who was rated as 'markedly downplaying/looking on the brightside' when she reported:

> I wish everything was alright, but it's not and I can't change that. So, I have to make the best of it. I feel that it could have been an awful lot worse. I feel that we're very, very lucky, because he could have all those health problems which he hasn't got. He's a very good baby, he sleeps, no trouble. Just physically he's low. He's not 100%, but whose perfect?

Another woman coped with her financial difficulty following an event of husband loss of overtime work which had supplemented their income:

> We just counted ourselves lucky that we actually had a roof over our heads and that the gas wasn't cut off, and the kids were alright and we were alright and Gerry had a job. I always thought Chris (friend) was in a far worse position than I was, homeless for a while and I thought 'I could be like that and with two children' which would be so much worse.

The presence or absence of support at the time of the crisis was also of significance in relation to onset of depression. The presence of crisis support related to lower rates of depression and was thus protective. Conversely, lack of support from a core tie (friend/close other) at the time of the crisis increased risk of depression. This particularly affected those who were 'let down' – that is, for those who did not receive the support they might have expected. This could be due to the support figure no longer being available (e.g. moved away) or in some instances because the crisis involved the support figure (e.g. death of mother who had been a confidant or breakdown in a previously confiding partner relationship).

However, it could also involve negative response from the support figure with hurtful and rejecting comments. Such let-down experiences were particularly harmful in increasing depression risk.

An example of good crisis support involves the following, when the respondent went into hospital for a routine operation and suffered a thrombosis leading to a five-week hospital stay. Her support figure was her close friend Jean:

> I told my friend Jean everything about the health problem – I always share my problems with her. She was extremely helpful. She actually took my daughter to stay with her and also helped my husband out with shopping, and household tasks. Jean was very supportive emotionally, reassuring me, even though she does have her own problems.

An example of lack of crisis support due to negative response (thus 'let-down') was reported by a woman who has been unable to get pregnant having a history of miscarriages and who then learns that her current pregnancy is ectopic and she requires a termination. Whilst she confided in her partner, she found it unhelpful:

> I've talked to him, cried with him a few times. But I can't really describe all my feelings about it. He does understand me wanting a baby. He gets emotional about it too. But it has gone on so long he just gets a bit fed up with me now.... gets a bit childish says things like "I might as well leave him".... stuff like that. That is what he said straight after the termination. I think he's tired of the whole process. It didn't help me when I was so upset. I think he's just switched off to me....

Figure 7.4 shows among vulnerable women studied in the Islington study (study 3, Appendix 1), who had a severe life event, the impact of crisis support from a friend or close other reduced risk of depression. Thus, all women represented in Figure 7.4 had either NES or negative elements in relationships as measured the year before, then had a severe life event and the graph shows those with and without crisis support and with and without poor coping at the time of the severe event. It can be seen that the lowest rates of depression occur where crisis support is present (the two right-hand columns). This holds even for those with poor coping (self-blame, pessimism or denial) where 13% became depressed, but for those with good coping, only 3% became depressed. This is significantly lower than the rates where lack of crisis support occurs (69% who also had poor coping and 25% with good coping). Thus, the worst scenario is for lack of crisis support and negative cognitive coping but crisis support plays a crucial role in protecting against depression. This is shown for women already known to be vulnerable. These are the types of findings that can usefully inform interventions given it is almost never too late in the process to provide support to avert symptoms.

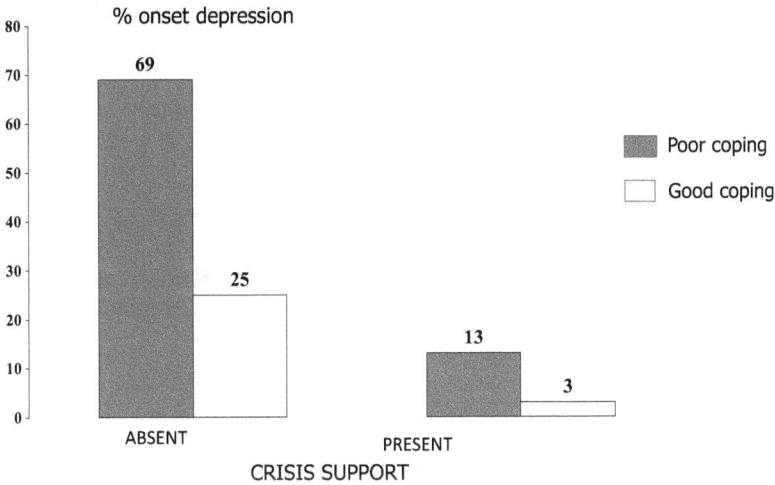

Figure 7.4 Crisis support, coping and depression.

The psychosocial life event model and interventions

The next section will look at psychosocial interventions as applied to the life event – depression model as outlined in this book. The following chapter (8) will outline interventions related to vulnerability. Whilst not aiming to be a fully comprehensive review of interventions, it will illustrate those most closely aligned to the model presented. It will also focus on adult interventions and therapies rather than those in childhood or adolescence. Nor will it outline those with parent–child or parenting focus which can be found elsewhere (Bifulco & Thomas, 2012). The interventions outlined here will be those which focus on life events and coping/crisis support categories (see Figure 7.5).

Psychosocial interventions for depression are very varied; at their most general, they comprise interpersonal (e.g. befriending) or informational (psychoeducational) strategies that target a range of risk factors with the aim of improving functioning or wellbeing. They can include psychotherapy approaches, community-based interventions, vocational rehabilitation, peer support through self-help and integrated care. These can be delivered in individual, family and group settings or via computer by a number of providers, including not only psychologists and psychiatrists but also social workers and community workers. Additionally, they can comprise standalone treatments, used together or combined with other approaches such as medicine (Institute of Medicine., 2015).

There is a robust evidence base for the effectiveness of psychosocial interventions in treating psychological disorder (NICE, 2009), yet implementation of evidence-based practice remains inconsistent, relying on local priorities, expertise availability and resources in the UK (Brooker & Brabban, 2004) and

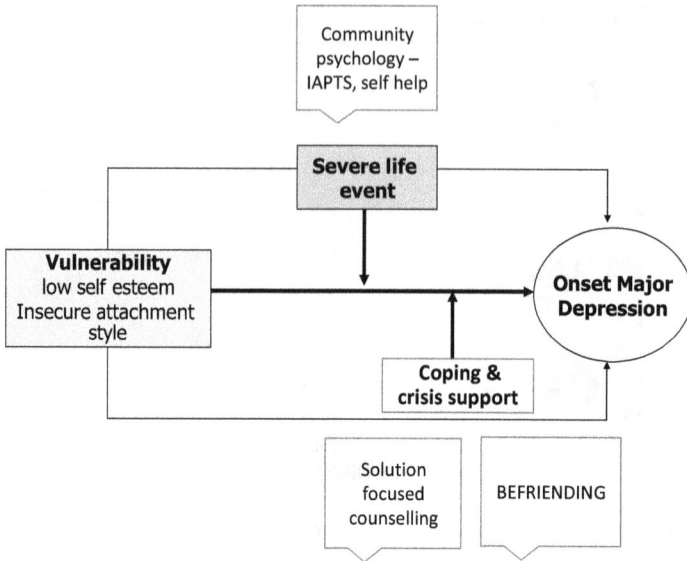

Figure 7.5 Interventions related to life events and coping.

USA (Institute of Medicine., 2015). Training of mental health workers can also be lacking, especially concerning the expertise on socio-environmental stress. Provision planned for wider access of psychosocial interventions to clients on a larger scale is described below. This is to tackle the social origins of disorder on a wider preventative scale and to increase the potential workforce of therapists.

Improving access to psychological therapies (IAPT)

Following Layard's exposition of rates of emotional disorder in the population, IAPT was instigated as a means of developing a skilled workforce of CBT practitioners without requiring an extended workforce of psychiatrists or clinical psychologists (Layard, 2006).

The IAPT programme began in 2008 to transform the treatment of adult depression and anxiety disorders in England.[1] IAPT is recognised as a very ambitious programme of talking therapies with more than one million people accessing it in a year to overcome their depression and anxiety and better manage their mental health. IAPT has also now increased the range of therapies (in addition to CBT) including counselling, couples therapy, interpersonal psychotherapy and brief psychodynamic therapy. The aim is to increase National Health Service (NHS) provision by an additional 380,000 individuals per year to reach 1.9 million by 2023–2024.

IAPT services are characterised by the following:

- **Evidence-based psychological therapies:** The therapy is delivered by fully trained and accredited practitioners, matched to the mental health problem and its intensity and duration designed to optimise outcomes. These are integrated with physical health pathways.
- **Routine outcome monitoring:** The person having therapy and the clinician offering it have up-to-date information on an individual's progress for a shared approach to the goals of therapy and transparency in service performance.
- **Regular and outcome-focused supervision:** Practitioners are supported to continuously improve and deliver high-quality care.

NHS England is working with NICE to support a new digitally enabled therapy assessment programme.[2] This will enable up to 14 digital therapy products to be accessed by 2020 to expand the provision of psychological therapies. These are currently undergoing testing. Digitally enabled therapy is provided online or through mobile applications, with the support of a therapist. There is evidence to show that these therapies can achieve comparable outcomes to face-to-face therapy, when the same content is delivered in an online format which allows much of the learning to be achieved through patient self-study, reinforced and supported by a suitably trained therapist (Andersson & Cuijpers, 2008; Rochlen, Zack, & Speyer, 2004). Indeed, this trend in treatment to reduce cost and widen access could fit well with online assessment measures such as provided by CLEAR. To date, these have not been combined to form an effective ongoing assessment and treatment process to apply to large numbers of individuals either at risk of emotional disorder or currently undergoing such disorder.

There have been problems identified with the IAPT approach. Operational and impact problems have been such that many local IAPT services, early in the development of the scheme, did not achieve a 50% recovery rate and that sessions are noted as costing three times more to fund than planned. Also, a high dropout rate was observed, and finally, fewer than half of the clinical commissioning groups met the target for the number of people accessing talking therapies (in 2017). One of the major issues in the future will be funding and resources to meet demand (especially now in the context of the financial and mental health impact of Covid-19). This involves practitioners often facing a higher level of psychological need and complex disorder than expected or training can facilitate, often due to lack of availability of more acute services. It also provides additional strain for practitioners working under pressure due to lack of intense supervision (Binnie, 2015, 2018; Watts, 2016). However, it also has many advocates who see it as fulfilling a much needed service (Clark, 2018).

Coping and crisis support interventions

Some of the interventions already described focus on life event crises. For example, around partner break up, bereavement and interpersonal difficulties. However, certain counselling approaches, as well as self-help groups, are focused on coping with particular crises as a relatively short-term intervention. Here, we will illustrate some particular crisis intervention approaches.

Solution-focused therapy

Solution-focused therapy is a humanistic approach which utilises a brief approach to finding solutions to the problems clients' have.[3] It contrasts a solution-focused approach with that of problem-solving, with an emphasis on strengths and the achievement of goals in a strictly time-limited approach (Trepper, Dolan, McCollum, & Nelson, 2006). It was developed in the late 1970s by Steve de Shazer and Insoo Kim Berg on seven basic principles (de Shazer et al., 1986):

- Change is both constant and certain
- Clients must want to change
- Clients are the experts and outline their own goals
- Clients have resources and their own strengths to solve and overcome their problems
- Therapy is short term
- Emphasis is on what is changeable and possible
- Focus on the future – history is not essential.

It therefore enhances the individual's own skills and resources and applies them to the problem at hand. It has been well evaluated (Schmit, Schmit, & Lenz, 2016), with effectiveness tested for treating symptoms of emotional disorders with youth and adults across 26 studies. Separate meta-analytic procedures yielded modest effect sizes. In addition, its advantages include its brevity (Rothwell, 2005) and its focus on resiliency (Gray & Wilker, 2008). Solution-focused therapy also focuses on what has gone well in recent attempts to cope with difficult issues, problems or life events. As such, it helps to align the client with noticing their strengths, utilising resources and identifying positive change. This maybe helpful for recognising positive life events for those with attachment issues.

Befriending and crisis support

Befriending is a means of providing social support to those who lack it. It has been suggested that a significant proportion of people present with distress because of social, physical and economic problems and that they may benefit from social interventions that do not medicalise their difficulties. Given the significant literature suggesting that social support affects the onset, course and outcome of depression and that individuals with distress appreciate emotional and social support, it is fitting that interventions should seek to address these issues (Dean & Goodlad, 1998). One way of providing social support is through befriending, defined as:

> a relationship between two or more individuals which is initiated, supported and monitored by an agency that has defined one or more parties as likely to benefit. Ideally the relationship is non-judgemental, mutual, and purposeful, and there is a commitment over time.

It can also be especially attuned to bereavement experiences (Harris, 2006).

Befriending is usually provided by volunteers with some basic training in how to provide effective social support and who meet up regularly with the individual in need (Harris, 2006). This approach, advocated by Tirril Harris, has been tested within the research model described in this book (Harris, Brown, & Robinson, 1999a, 1999b). A study by the Bedford Square team tested a befriending intervention with a sample of chronically depressed women (op cit). Befriending was found to have a significant effect on remission in those with chronic depression. Further analysis showed that the presence of fresh start experiences, absence of new severe stressors and secure attachment style were important predictors of remission.

A systematic review of befriending for depression was undertaken (Mead, Lester, Chew-Graham, Gask, & Bower, 2010) comprising 24 studies of randomised trials of interventions focused on providing emotional support to individuals in the community, usually with a 'treatment as usual' comparison group. Befriending was defined as an intervention that 'introduces the client to one or more individuals whose main aim is to provide the client with additional social support through the development of an affirming, emotion-focused relationship over time'. The relationship should be established and monitored via an agency that has identified one or more parties as likely to benefit. The social support offered was primarily non-directive and emotional in nature. Studies in the review were excluded where informational, instrumental or appraisal support formed a key component of the intervention. Only befriending interventions delivered on an individual basis (either in person or via the telephone or internet) were included. 'Befrienders' could be untrained lay persons or professionals qualified in relationship-based interventions. Where the befriender was a trained professional, great attention was paid to ensure that the befriending actions were focused on developing a non-directive, emotion-focused relationship. Studies where the 'befriender' was a member of the client's existing social or care provider network (e.g. family member, caseworker, general practitioner) were excluded. The review found that compared with usual care or no treatment, befriending had a modest but significant effect on depressive symptoms in the short term and long term. Befriending was however less effective than CBT with adolescents and in medication-resistant individuals with schizophrenia and was less effective than nurse cognitive–behavioural problem-solving in carers of people with dementia.

Provision of emotional support through befriending in the NHS could therefore have many advantages for individuals, mental health services and the wider health economy. It could, for example, extend patient choice within the lower levels of the recommended 'stepped care' model for depression and provide a less-medicalised approach to emotional distress. It could also offer a preventative strategy for individuals at risk of developing psychological disorder in line with the major UK policy focus on health prevention throughout the NHS. Less costly and onerous staff training requirements could improve both implementation and access to treatment, especially if combined with a telephone-based system such as those being developed in other mental health services. Low cost might make such an intervention more feasible in low-income countries and those where the proportion of health budget spending on mental health is relatively small. There are also a large number of peer-led or peer-supported interventions involving people with lived experience of mental health issues. This has implications for some of the interventions outlined, for example, befriending. Thus, people who have experienced similar life events or difficulties, along with psychological disorders, maybe able to offer support and solutions based in their own experiences. This may be viewed as less stigmatising by the recipients. Also, some interventions are interestingly combining peer-led approaches with online interventions (Pfeiffer et al., 2020).

Clinical implications of positive events

A tailored focus on the type of crisis experienced, by accurately mapping different individual vulnerabilities, could tailor intervention or preventative strategies with ever greater precision. This could make more informed clinical judgements about the most appropriate treatment paths. This approach is beginning to be employed in the field of 'precision psychiatry', which comes from the broader field of precision medicine. The latter is an emerging medical approach for treating and preventing physical disease which takes into account individual differences in genes, environment or lifestyle, thus allowing doctors and researchers to more accurately predict which treatment and prevention strategies will work for which people. This approach could similarly be applied to a more precise clinical psychological approach.

For instance, one of the research projects conducted by the Bedford Square team (the Coping project, study 5, Appendix 1) was able to select women by questionnaire from GP surgery lists, who all had vulnerability and yet were free from depression, and followed them up at four monthly intervals over 18 months. In this group, there was more than a four-fold higher rate of new depression (45%) than expected from a representative group (10%) living in the same area (Bifulco et al., 1998). Thus, it was possible to predict over a four-fold increase in depression risk in a relatively short period of time. Yet all were screened fairly simply by questionnaire (Vulnerability to Depression Questionnaire – VDQ) (Moran, Bifulco, Ball, & Campbell, 2001) and would be an appropriate group to select for potential preventative work. In particular, to focus an intervention first on presenting vulnerability and also on building capacity for crisis coping and support. This would provide greater precision to such intervention.

The research presented regarding positive events raises issues for clinicians. Individual differences are implicated in differing responses to positive experiences. This is important because individuals with depression are often encouraged to undertake behavioural activation, whereby they engage in activities and events that they are likely to enjoy. This to reengage them with roles and relationships and lessen helplessness and hopelessness. However, individuals with low self-esteem and poor support may derive less enhancement from experiencing positive events and those with low self-esteem can actually begin to feel worse.

Therefore, as discussed in the next chapter, therapy needs to target self-esteem as well as core beliefs and attitudes around positive experiences in order to maximise the benefits from these sorts of interventions and increase general responsiveness to the external environment.

Notes

1 https://www.england.nhs.uk/mental-health/adults/iapt/
2 https://www.nice.org.uk/about/what-we-do/our-programmes/nice-advice/iapt
3 https://www.counselling-directory.org.uk/solution-focused-brief-therapy.html

8 Positive events and wellbeing

Subjective wellbeing involves a person's positive cognitive (thinking) and affective (feeling) evaluations of their life. This includes a sense of optimism and life satisfaction together with feelings of pleasure and happiness. It includes both *hedonic* perspectives, that of maximising pleasure and minimising pain, and *eudemonic* perspectives, involving self-realisation and attaining meaning in life. Both are relevant to good quality of life and feelings of wellbeing. Both can be increased by experiencing events which are highly positive.

Unlike clinical conditions, subjective wellbeing is commonly measured by questionnaire, specifically with items reflecting the hedonic aspects of life satisfaction, optimism and positive mood and feelings. An example is the Warwick-Edinburgh Mental Wellbeing Scale (WEMWBS) (Tennant et al., 2007) which consists of 14 positively worded items regarding thoughts and feelings over the previous two weeks. It includes feelings of optimism ('I've been feeling optimistic about the future'), being instrumental ('I've been feeling useful'), sociability ('I've been feeling interested in other people'), good functioning ('I've been thinking clearly') and self-esteem ('I've been feeling good about myself'). The scale has published defined cut-offs for high, moderate and low wellbeing. Thus, high scores can be utilised to evidence a particularly good state of wellbeing. Whilst less episodic than disorders such as depression, wellbeing is associated with more enduring positive personal characteristics and acknowledged as open to change. It is also associated with positive relationships and beliefs about self, others and the future – effectively a positive rather than negative cognitive triad (Seligman, 2011). This indication of psychological robustness can be seen as the opposite side of the coin to vulnerability.

Psychosocial models of wellbeing can potentially be expanded and improved by the inclusion of positive life events. Therefore, just as a vulnerability-provoking agent model can explain onset of depression, we need to consider if the obverse applies – that markers of prior psychological robustness can interact with positive events to impact on increasing wellbeing. This chapter further explores characteristics of positive life events, including those stabilising and enhancing to a person's life in relation to wellbeing. We will demonstrate how these characteristics can be added to our conceptual model to help us understand what underpins positive life events and how they impact the four underlying psychological needs of attachment, security, identity and achievement to increase wellbeing.

However, just as there is evidence to suggest that not all people who experience negative life events will develop depression, not all people who experience positive life events will have a concomitant increase in wellbeing (Lyubomirsky & Tucker, 1998). Wellbeing, unlike depression, is not really episodic, but is prone to fluctuation over time. Thus, instead of one critical event creating an 'onset' as with depression, it seems that the effects of positive life events can accumulate to enhance wellbeing (Gomez, Krings, Bangerter, & Grob, 2009). Additionally, there is evidence that experiencing one positive life event increases the likelihood of subsequent positive life events occurring, and in the absence of negative life events, creating a cumulative effect on wellbeing (Young, Machell, Kashdan, & Westwater, 2018). In fact, when compared to the individual's average number of life events, the more life events experienced over a two-year period, the greater the increase (if positive events) or decrease (if negative events) in life satisfaction (Headey, 2006). Therefore, the sequencing of positive and negative events over time appears to be important for longer-term wellbeing.

To explore a positive model involving robustness, we examine secure attachment style as a predisposing factor. Secure attachment style is the normative attachment style, the most common in normal populations, and the most functional. It involves flexibility in relating to close others, having ability to give and seek help and to build close confiding attachments (Bowlby, 1988). It is related to benign childhood experience, good adult support, fewer severe life events and low adversity, together with lower rates of psychological disorder (Bifulco & Thomas, 2012). It also relates to more sophisticated coping with stressors (Mikulincer, Gillath, & Shaver, 2002). As with other attachment styles, it is relatively enduring but may change under duress (Cozzarelli, Karafa, Collins, & Tagler, 2003).

There are numerous measures of attachment style but only two established interviews – the Attachment Style Interview (ASI) (Bifulco & Thomas, 2012) described earlier and also the Adult Attachment Interview (AAI) (George, Kaplan, & Main, 1984). There are however many self-report questionnaires (Stein, Jacobs, Ferguson, Allen, & Fonagy, 1998). We have referred earlier to the Vulnerable Attachment Style Questionnaire (VASQ) which is validated against the ASI (Bifulco, Mahon, Kwon, Moran, & Jacobs, 2003) and is described in relation to CLEAR and depression (Bifulco, Kagan, et al., 2019). Findings from the ASI indicate secure attachment style is *inversely* related to negative self-esteem (Bifulco, Moran, Ball, & Lillie, 2002), childhood adversity and to onset of depression (Bifulco, Moran, Ball, & Bernazzani, 2002). We will seek to examine the relationship of secure attachment style to positive life events and wellbeing later in this chapter.

Model of positive event-related need (ASIA)

In a previous chapter, the parallels between features of severe events which increased depression risk and the four-fold basic needs models were presented. The model explained the important negative dimensions of life events tied to key needs. Below we expand this model by outlining how the positive dimensions can also be tied to these fundamental areas.

Attachment – being loved

Positive attachment events focus on relationships, their restoration following events such as someone moving closer to live, a reconciliation after an argument or the formation of a new relationship. In terms of predisposing attachment style, the effects of secure attachment on positive functioning have had less focus in the research literature than the impacts of insecure style on disorder. The distinctions between types of insecure style have had a large focus in relating to different behaviours and risks for disorder (Bifulco & Thomas, 2012). Yet secure attachment is not simply the 'residual' style, but the most highly functioning, and it behoves us to understand the flexibility and adaptability it bestows. There is evidence that how people perceive, interpret and think about life events is linked to their general happiness (Lyubomirsky & Ross, 1999; Lyubomirsky & Tucker, 1998), and there is indication that the way positive events are processed differs as a product of attachment. Certainly, insecurely attached individuals are less able to access memories of positive events (Mikulincer, 1998) and underestimate how good they felt after positive experiences (Gentzler & Kerns, 2006) and minimise positive experiences. Securely attached individuals savour and appreciate positive experiences (Gentzler, Kerns, & Keener, 2010; Gentzler, Ramsey, Yi, Palmer, & Morey, 2014). This suggests that insecurely attached individuals are not able to take advantage of positive life events and respond in the same way that securely attached individuals do. Individuals with insecure styles additionally have lower levels of social support and are less able to use close others to help regulate their emotions, avoiding real intimacy within relationships. In contrast, securely attached individuals often rely on support-seeking strategies to aid their coping with events and reduce negative emotion created. It is possible that individuals who cannot effectively use social support are more reliant on positive life changes to regulate their mood. Positive life events are more strongly associated with time to remission in those with small available networks than those who tend to withdraw in the face of problems (Oldehinkel, Ormel, & Neeleman, 2000). Thus, secure attachment style, support and positive events appear to have a mutual influence on each other for wellbeing.

Security – being safe

Security events increase an individual's feelings of being safe, whether this is due to increase in predictability and stability (e.g. routinisation events such as returning to work after a sickness break), increased commitment and permanence (e.g. anchoring events such as getting married or receiving a permanent work contract) or bestowing a sense of hope after difficulty and a reduction in the potential for harm (e.g. relief events such as receiving medication for a chronic condition with fewer side effects). In this way, security tends to be related to events that give an increased ability to meet such needs whether material or relational as well as the reduction of chronic difficulties and long-term problems which threaten a sense of safety.

As previously discussed, studies show that a reduction in a chronic difficulty increases the probability of remission in depression and anxiety, separately from the occurrence of a positive life event (Harris, Brown, & Robinson, 1999b; Leenstra, Ormel, & Giel, 1995; Ronalds, Creed, Stone, Webb, & Tomenson, 1997). This holds across a variety of clinical disorders (Neeleman, Oldehinkel, & Ormel, 2003). To give a specific example, a study by Choi and Marks investigated reciprocal relationships between marital conflict and depression over a 15-year period (Choi & Marks, 2008). They found a feedback loop between fluctuations in a chronic difficulty (in this case marital conflict) and depressive symptoms. A parallel view of positive security would indicate time lags between marital closeness and satisfaction and wellbeing, expected to increase with advancing age. Given the association of positive events with attachment security and confiding relationships, it can be deduced that such positive feedback loops are also maintained. Thus, reductions in difficulties by positive events which confer increased stability in life can reduce symptoms of disorder and potentially increase wellbeing.

Identity – belonging and self-esteem

Identity, self-esteem and belongingness are closely connected. A sociometer theory of self-esteem theorises that self-esteem is a measure of an individual's social connectedness (Leary, 2012). This is based on the idea that people have an innate need to form and maintain social bonds, and their self-esteem tells them how well they are doing in this regard. Events that involve being accepted or included by others, such as a refugee who gains citizenship or a foster child being officially adopted, are likely to increase feelings of belonging whether on a community or individual basis and will therefore raise self-esteem. Events which feature social rejection and exclusion will be related to lowered self-esteem. However, not all events which raise and lower self-esteem involve actual changes to an individual's level of belonging. Certainly, achievement events are linked to identity and increased self-esteem in their own right. For example, a lawyer who gets a promotion or a writer who wins a literary competition is likely to help confirm that individual's identity in relation to those roles. Nevertheless, achievement may also be related to social acceptance, even if more obliquely; events which feature task failures such as a demotion or a failed audition are more likely to be linked to a fear or perception of social rejection in people with low self-esteem (Baldwin & Sinclair, 1996).

As discussed earlier, positive events often precede remission from anxiety and depression. However, they do not precede all remissions, and people who experience positive events can also remain ill. Other factors change the effect of positive events and their ability to influence mental health. As described earlier, positive self-esteem (PES) is one of the factors that influence whether people benefit from positive life events. Interestingly, positive life events can sometimes detrimentally affect the health of those with negative self-esteem, this deriving from an identity disruption model of stress. This theory holds that an accumulation of life events that are inconsistent with the self-concept leads to physical illness (Brown & McGill, 1989); thus, an accumulation of positive life events that are inconsistent with an individual's negative self-concept has been found to lead to physical illness due to the identity disturbance caused. For example, a student who sees themselves as poor academically may have that self-image disrupted by an academic award creating uncertainty around concepts of the self and possible ill-health as a consequence. Similarly, it has been found that those with low self-esteem respond differently to achievement events, with these being more aversive than for people with high self-esteem as it heightens feelings of anxiety (Wood, Heimpel, Newby-Clark, & Ross, 2005). Thus, increasing self-esteem is shown as critical to individuals benefiting from positive events in increasing wellbeing.

Achievement – having success

Achievement relates to goal attainment, success and enhanced status. A positive event in this domain would be, for example, after working overtime for several months, an individual achieves a promotion with more responsibility and a greater salary. Achievement events and related positive emotion have been linked to the aspect of subjective wellbeing that concerns the meaning of life (Machell, Kashdan, Short, & Nezlek, 2015). This has generally focused on global meaning judgements but can also encompass meaning in daily life. For example, a study by Machell and colleagues of college students examined how their daily experiences influenced their perceived sense of meaning on a daily basis (Machell et al., 2015). Daily social and achievement events, daily positive and negative affect and daily meaning in life were examined with the possible moderating influence of depressive symptoms. Positive daily social and achievement events were related to greater daily meaning, above and beyond the contributions of daily positive and negative affect. Negative social and achievement events were related to less daily meaning, and negative achievement events co-varied with daily meaning above and beyond positive and negative affect. Depression moderated the relationships between positive events and meaning, such that people who reported more depressive symptoms had greater increases in daily meaning in response to positive social and achievement events than individuals who reported fewer symptoms. These findings suggest the important role that daily events may play in fluctuations in people's affective experiences and sense of meaning in life. Whilst potentially taking a lower threshold of what constitutes events in daily life, this study indicates that positive events can lead to greater increases in meaning for those with depression, presumably given a lower baseline with more potential for increase.

However, as discussed earlier, not all positive events have beneficial impacts, particularly for those with vulnerability, including those that involve goal attainment. Success events have been found to precede manic symptoms (Johnson et al., 2008) with confidence becoming unrealistically high in response to achievement. Potentially, the increased confidence spurs on greater activity related to goal pursuit, and this increased activity in turn may intensify goal pursuit, sleep loss and other processes thought to be risk factors for mania. This shows a potential downside to positive events in some individuals who are vulnerable. However, for those with more positive outlooks on life, achievement events can potentially increase wellbeing.

Testing positive events and wellbeing

In order to test whether positive events can increase levels of wellbeing, the online CLEAR project described earlier (see study 11, Appendix 1) examined positive life events in relation to a questionnaire measure of wellbeing. Following prior LEDS analysis, positive features of events were combined into two indices (see Figure 8.1). Here, the stabilising events were close to the prior study definitions of anchoring, but the enhancing events utilised somewhat different labels with 'reconciliation' and 'restoration' rather than 'fresh start' as a label. These are summarised below and then further discussed.

Reconciliation signifies an increase in the quality of relationships following a period of separation, conflict or coldness. Reconciliation events would, for example, include siblings who meet to mend their relationship after a period of conflict. Although reconciliation is often concerned with improved attachments, it can touch on other basic needs. For example, feuding business partners who reconcile in order to work together to save their company may also increase feelings of security because their company is less likely to fail. This event may also affect achievement if the fortunes of their company begin to turn around with public recognition of success. Another example might be parents who have been going through a bitter divorce, meeting to reconcile and jointly find a strategy to deal with their child's problem. As well as impacting on attachment, this might enhance their role identity as parents. Restoration occurs when something that was lost is restored. Examples include when an individual gets a better job after being

---

Stability events - one ofthe following:

- Anchoring - grounding events (e.g. finding secure accommodation; permanent job).
- Routinising - increases stability of predictable routines.
- Relief - event reduces prior level of problem (health improvement).

Enhancing events - one ofthe following:

- Reconciliation - making up after separation due to conflict/coldness.
- Restoration - something lost restored e.g.work role reinstated; relationship resumed after absence.
- Enhancing self-image – e.g.winning prize; promotion; appearance after plastic surgery.

Figure 8.1 CLEAR project positive event definitions.

made unemployed or a person receives from the police their stolen bag complete with bank cards, money and phone. Or when important documents are recovered on a computer after being corrupted. Restoration events can affect any of the four basic needs depending on what is being restored.

Examples of positive events linked to need

Attachment: Someone who emigrated returns home restoring lost relationships (Restoration); a sister resumes a relationship after a period of conflict and loss of contact (Reconciliation).

Security: Someone finds a house after being made homeless restoring their feeling of safety and stability (Anchoring).

Identity: After a trial separation, a couple reunite restoring their roles as husband and wife (Restoration); a trainee cadet becoming a police officer (Goal Achievement); improving body image through intervention, such as a change to disfigurement after plastic surgery (Self-image enhancement).

Achievement: After losing out on one round of bidding for a lucrative contract, a company's application is successful elsewhere (Goal Achievement).

In the CLEAR project, positivity was queried for every event reported and self-rated on a 4-point scale for level of positivity. Further characteristics were presented in a checklist fashion for all events, but only included in the analysis for events identified as positive (at 'marked' or 'moderate' level of positivity) (Spence, Kagan, et al., in submission). Other characteristics included as possible robustness were the presence of close confidants and secure attachment style as measured by the VASQ (Bifulco, Mahon, et al., 2003). Wellbeing was assessed by the Warwick Edinburgh Mental Wellbeing Scale described earlier in this chapter.

Positive events were prevalent in the CLEAR sample, with just under half the 236 people studied (48%) having experienced at least one in the prior 12 months and 22% having two or more. A third of the sample had a stabilising event and 22% had an enhancing positive event. Positive events were significantly related to wellbeing score ($r = 0.12$, $p < 0.01$). Nine per cent of the sample had high wellbeing, and this was more common in the midlife control group (21%) with rates of only 4% in the prior clinical group and 5% in the student group ($p < 0.0001$). There was no difference in rates of having at least one positive event by study group. However, the student group had higher rates of stabilising and enhancing events, despite lower wellbeing (Spence, Kagan, et al., in submission) (see Figure 8.2). This is perhaps explained by these events emerging out of periods of difficulty.

Somewhat contradictory findings occurred when age was examined as a variable in the sample as a whole. Younger individuals were significantly more likely to have experienced a positive event with more stabilising features ($r = -0.13$, $p < 0.05$), but this did not hold for enhancing features ($r = -0.08$, $p = 0.09$). Wellbeing, however, increased with age ($r = 0.23$, $p < 0.01$) and was associated with having more positive life events ($r = 0.12$, $p < 0.01$) and more close confiding relationships ($r = 0.11$, $p < 0.01$) (Spence, Kagan, et al., in submission). Thus, the young in the sample do experience positive events, but also have less wellbeing.

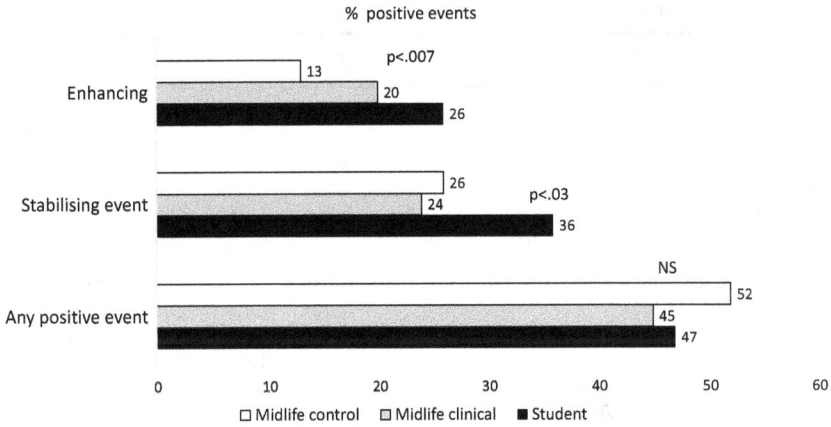

% positive events

Figure 8.2 Positive events in CLEAR project by group.

Secure attachment style was examined in a model looking at positive life events and wellbeing. This model of robustness was confirmed with secure attachment style related to positive events ($r = 0.14$, $p < 0.01$) and to wellbeing ($r = 0.57$, $p < 0.01$). An ANOVA statistic showed that individuals with a secure attachment style had significantly higher wellbeing ($F(1, 486) = 122.81$, $p < 0.001$), reported significantly more positive events ($F(1, 486) = 4.47$, $p = 0.04$), had more close relationships ($F(1, 486) = 17.36$, $p < 0.001$) and higher levels of confiding ($F(1, 486) = 38.59$, $p < 0.001$).

Hierarchical multiple regression indicated a significant interaction between secure attachment style, positive life events and wellbeing (see Table 8.1). This reflects the third step in a hierarchical multiple regression model and shows the interaction between positive life events and secure attachment style.

Utilising the total score for wellbeing, multiple regression demonstrated that experiencing a positive event tended to increase the wellbeing score by 0.66 points on the scale, whilst on average, individuals with a secure attachment style scored approximately eight points higher on wellbeing. Attachment style and number of positive events remained significantly related to wellbeing when controlling for levels of confiding and the number of close others. The interaction between attachment style and positive events was significant, meaning that the increase in wellbeing after experiencing a positive event was dependent on secure attachment style. An individual with a secure attachment style who had experienced an average number of positive events should expect to score approximately 49 on wellbeing, whilst an insecurely attached individual would expect to score about 42. For every positive event experienced, a securely attached individual's wellbeing score increased by 1.28 points, while an insecurely attached individual's score only increased by 0.02 (see Figure 8.3). Both the models explained about 22% of the variance in wellbeing.

Table 8.1 Final model of positive life events and insecure attachment on wellbeing.

Step 3[c]	B	(s.e.)	β	T
Hierarchical multiple regression				
Constant	37.45*	1.18		31.77
Total positive events	0.03	0.40	0.00	0.08
Secure attachment style	5.74*	1.06	0.29	5.42
Total positive events * secure attachment	1.15**	0.58	0.12	1.97
Confiding	−0.66	0.66	−0.06	−1.01
People close	0.73	0.38	0.11	1.93
Age	0.29*	0.04	0.57	6.60
Gender	1.44	0.97	0.06	1.48
Group	−7.48*	1.04	−0.57	−7.19

*p < 0.001, **p < 0.05, [c]R^2 = 0.299.

It was shown in an earlier chapter that students in the CLEAR project had higher rates of severe life events than the midlife participants, so it is interesting that they also have higher rates of positive events involving stabilising and enhancing features. However, for many, it related to the ending of precarious negative situations (e.g. financial worries, study difficulties). Perhaps, this reflects the fact that younger individuals as students often experience periods of flux and uncertainty associated with this life stage; with students in the modern world with increased access to universities through loan schemes suffering from having fewer material resources with which to study. They appear to experience higher rates of both negative and positive events – thus, more events overall. Yet the students also had significantly lower wellbeing, with high rates of depression, suggesting that positive events did not exert a beneficial effect. The issue of why some individuals can respond to positive experiences with positive affect and others not, has already been discussed in relation to vulnerable versus robust predisposing characteristics. Secure attachment style is identified as a key factor for creating conditions for the valuing of positive events. This is also known to be associated with physiological responsivity and cognitive receptiveness and will be examined further below.

In the CLEAR study, individuals with a secure attachment style had significantly higher wellbeing and reported significantly more positive events. Additionally, there was a significant interaction between attachment style and positive events, with securely attached individuals experiencing a significantly greater increase in wellbeing after a positive life event. This suggests that in terms of subjective wellbeing, securely attached individuals are able to gain from positive life events in a way that insecurely attached individuals are not. The implication is that those with insecure attachment style are unable to appraise the positive and to respond with the relevant cognition or emotion. Affective responses can influence whether an event is judged as positive or negative (Young et al., 2018). Research demonstrates that individuals who make global, internal and stable attributions for recent positive events (i.e. the event reflects something that will be true over time,

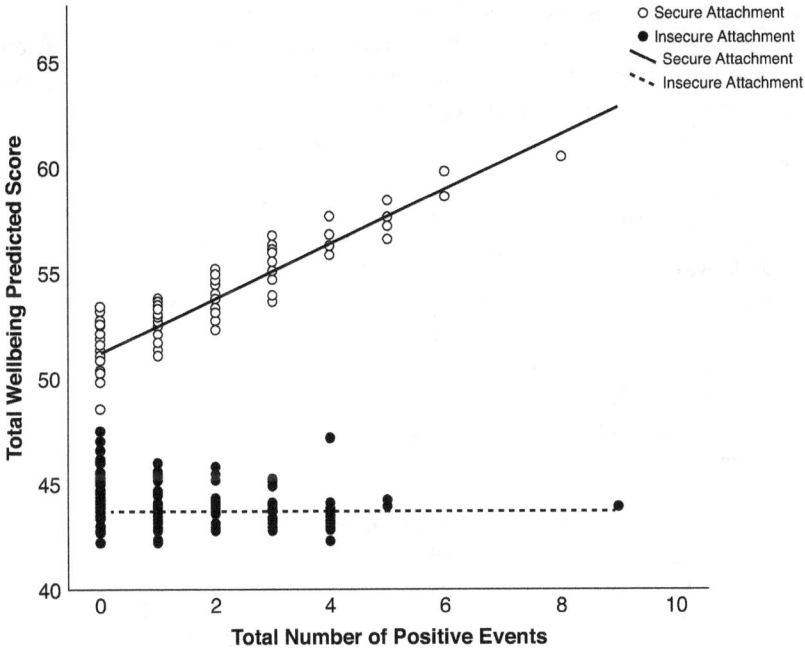

Figure 8.3 Predicted total wellbeing score by attachment style and number of positive events with fit lines added by attachment style.

is due to something about the individual and applies to many domains) show decreases in depressive symptom levels (Johnson, Han, Douglas, Johannet, & Russell, 1998). This does not hold for those with insecure styles, and Beckian negative schemata could be applied to explain this finding. This includes low self-esteem (Fuhr, Reitenbach, Kraemer, Hautzinger, & Meyer, 2017), hopelessness (Lavy & Littman-Ovadia, 2011) and fragility of happiness; the belief that happiness can cause bad things to happen and that when happiness is achieved, it will not last long (Joshanloo, 2018). In these scenarios, positive life events are construed differently, with suspicion and mistrust and thus not experienced as increasing wellbeing.

Positive event and wellbeing examples

Two examples are given here of positive events as associated with high levels of wellbeing. One is taken from the CLEAR student group and the other from the midlife sample.

Carla's case

Carla is a 19-year-old international student from Greece. She has just started her university marketing degree, and this is the reason she moved to the UK. She works part-time and has a boyfriend whom she has been dating for five months. Both her parents are in Greece, and she is close to both of them as well as her best friend Julia, with whom she has daily contact. She recently got a student loan so she could begin studying and went to her first-ever job interview to get a job to supplement her income. Carla moved into halls of residence shortly after arriving in the UK and that is where she met Julia and became close. She reported high wellbeing (WEMWBS = 65) and described four positive events over the course of 12 months.

1   Carla was pleased to receive her student loan as it made it possible for her to study abroad in the UK (Education, 1: marked positivity, stabilising).
2   She was also excited to be starting her university course in the UK, and she had no problems settling in and enjoys the course (Education, 2: moderate positivity, stabilising).
3   Carla went to a few job interviews; she had never had one before and reported feeling some anxiety before but she began to enjoy them and secured herself a part-time job (Work, 3: some positivity, stabilising).
4   Carla met someone when she started university, he became her boyfriend and this developed into a serious relationship which makes her happy (Partner, 2: moderate positivity, enhancing).

These events have the effect of adding to Carla's sense of achievement (her studies) as well as her social life (attachment) to add to the enjoyability of this new phase in her life.

Miranda's case

Miranda is a 54-year-old divorced accountant. She lives in a semi-detached house which she now owns outright. She has six children and lives with three of them. She recorded three of her grown children as being her confidants. Two of her sons are twins; during the year, they sat their GCSEs, and her daughter also gave birth to her first grandchild. It was a difficult birth, with the child not breathing at first, but after testing, they considered the baby to be fine and there have been no longer-term ramifications. Miranda reported high wellbeing (WEMWBS = 62) and three positive life events over the course of 12 months.

1   Her twin sons, Stewart and Robert, sat their GCSE exams; they both did very well getting good results after working hard. Miranda was pleased that they received similar results as this led to less tension in the house (Education, 2: moderate, enhancing).
2   Miranda has had a large mortgage with expensive repayments, but she finally managed to pay off the remainder and now owns her house outright (Finance, 1: marked positivity, stabilising).
3   Miranda's daughter had a baby, Rose; this was Miranda's first grandchild. The birth was difficult because Rose wasn't breathing at first but all tests

have come back fine and there have been no problems since (Children, 1: marked positivity, enhancing).

These events have the effect of adding to Miranda's sense of security in her middle-age (housing) as well as enhancing her attachment (through her new grandchild) and her identity (role enhancement) through her sons' achievement. (Note that the birth difficulties in relation to the grandchild means that the event could also have a threat rating.)

Adding to the model

Figure 8.4 illustrates how the positive events identified map on to the proposed model. Although the different event types can straddle more than one aspect, for ease, we have placed them where it seems most appropriate. Thus, positive self is linked to identity events, new roles and those which improve self-image; positive people is linked to attachment events and events that feature reconciliation or restoration; positive future is linked to achievement and fresh start events and events that include relief; and positive world is linked to stabilising events and events that involve anchoring characteristics.

Interventions to promote wellbeing

In this section, we consider interventions available to decrease vulnerability and promote wellbeing (see Figure 8.5). The vulnerability factors identified in this book are varied including those distal in childhood (neglect or abuse) or those

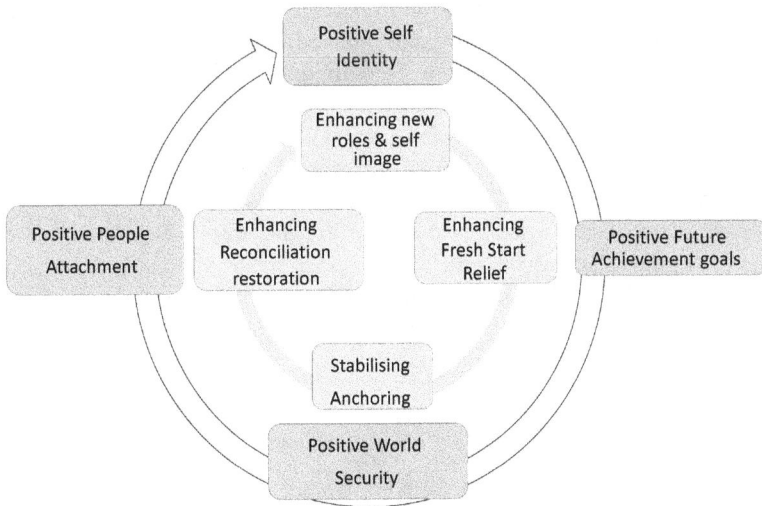

Figure 8.4 Model of needs, positive cognitive function and positive events.

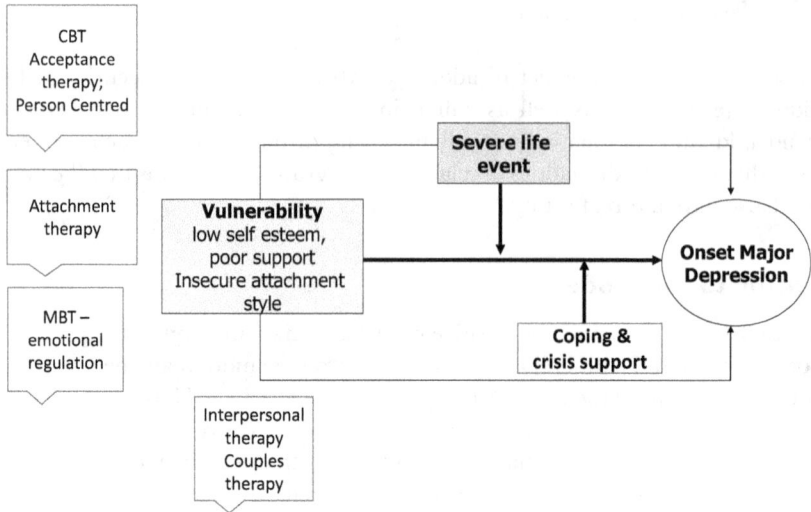

Figure 8.5 Interventions to tackle vulnerability.

biological (disrupted cortisol or genetic or epigenetic phenomena) as well as those proximal (including insecure attachment style, lack of support and low self-esteem). The genetic research has recommended a 'what works for whom' application of the understanding of genetic risk or resilience (Belsky & Van Ijzendoorn, 2015). Belsky and Van Ijzendoorn in editing a special edition of the 'Development and Psychopathology' journal looked at the genetic moderation of intervention efficacy (op cit). They refer to G × I (gene × intervention) as a follow up to G × E and note that this has been slower in developing. They focus on the differential genetic susceptibility hypothesis to tailor interventions to the person and indicate which will work best for whom. Thus, recognition that characteristics of individuals influence the efficacy of the intervention. This does of course raise issues of equity (who is allocated to what programme) but may well increase efficacy.

Additionally, for adults, childhood risks tend to be approached in terms of the proximal mediating risks of negative cognitions or attachment insecurity. Therefore, most psychological interventions are therapies which focus on ongoing adult cognitive-affective characteristics (such as negative self-evaluation) or interpersonal style, involving communication and conflict-resolution in relationships. This can encompass individual therapy, partner therapy or family therapy. These are described below.

Cognitive behaviour therapy – changing negative thinking

The most popularly approved therapy by psychologists due to the documented evidence-base is that of cognitive behaviour therapy (CBT) (Chu & Harrison, 2007). This has certain underpinning principles but can then be applied to a range of issues including anger-management, bereavement issues or trauma. Originally espoused by Aaron Beck, it is defined as a psycho-social intervention that aims to improve mental health.[1] It focuses on challenging and changing unhelpful cognitive distortions and behaviours, improving emotional regulation and the development of personal coping strategies that target solving current problems. Originally, it was designed to treat depression, but its uses have been expanded to include treatment of a number of other disorders, including anxiety. CBT includes a number of cognitive or behaviour psychotherapies that treat defined psychopathologies using evidence-based techniques and strategies.

The protocol as simply described on the NHS website states[2]:

- CBT is based on the concept that your thoughts, feelings, physical sensations and actions are interconnected and that negative thoughts and feelings can trap you in a vicious cycle.
- CBT aims to help you deal with overwhelming problems in a more positive way by breaking them down into smaller parts.
- A person is shown how to change these negative patterns to improve the way they feel.
- Unlike some other talking treatments, CBT deals with current problems rather than focussing on issues from the past.
- It looks for practice ways to improve a person's stage of mind on a daily basis.

CBT is considered to be one of the most effective evidence-based treatments (Chu & Harrison, 2007; Huguet et al., 2016) including with economic analysis (Kaltenthaler et al., 2006) and has been transferred to online versions with some success (Romero-Sanchiz et al., 2017). Criticisms have been detailed and countered (Gaudiano, 2011). These include the approach being overly mechanistic, too symptom-based, weakly associated with basic cognitive science or basic science in general, that the mechanisms of change are not well supported and that improvement often occurs before the cognitive intervention (op cit). However, a common criticism is also about its frugality – with NHS providing for only 10–12 sessions.

Acceptance and commitment therapy – changing negative feelings

Acceptance and commitment therapy (ACT) stems from traditional behaviour therapy and CBT (Hayes, Strosahl, & Wilson, 2011), but has a change in focus which de-emphasises the idea of something being wrong with the individual. Clients learn to stop avoiding, denying and struggling with their inner emotions and, instead, accept that these deeper feelings are appropriate responses to certain situations that should not prevent them from moving forward in their lives. With this understanding, clients begin to accept their issues and hardships and commit to making necessary changes in their behaviour, regardless of what is going on in their lives, and how they feel about it. In many ways, this accepts that the life events are really external stressors to contend with and that some of us are less well-equipped to deal with them due to early life hardships.

According to ACT's underlying theory, psychological disorders result from attempting to avoid a past experience; thus, a goal of treatment with ACT is to develop more accepting, mindful attitudes towards distressing memories and negative conditions rather than avoiding them. You learn to listen to the way you talk to yourself specifically about traumatic events, problematic relationships, physical limitations or other issues. You can then decide if an issue requires immediate action and change or if it can – or must – be accepted for what it is while you learn to make behavioural changes that can affect the situation. You may look at what hasn't worked for you in the past so that the therapist can help you stop repeating thought patterns and behaviours that are causing you more problems in the long run.

ACT addresses six core processes: acceptance, defusion, present moment awareness, self-as-context, values and committed action. The theory behind ACT is that it is often counterproductive to try to control painful emotions or psychological experiences because suppression of these feelings ultimately leads to more distress. ACT theorises that there are valid alternatives to trying to change the way you think, and these include mindful behaviour, attention to personal values and commitment to action. By taking steps to change their behaviour, while at the same time learning to accept their psychological experiences, clients can eventually change their attitude and emotional state.

Two systematic reviews, two randomised controlled trials and four non-randomised studies (NRS) assessed the clinical effectiveness of ACT for adult patients with trauma-related PTSD, anxiety or depression (Pohar & Argáez, 2017). The two systematic reviews included a limited number of case reports and 'poor-quality' studies, but found preliminary evidence supporting the use of ACT in PTSD. One of the two RCTs found favourable results for ACT combined with treatment as usual (TAU), compared to TAU alone in survivors of interpersonal trauma. Also, ACT has been reported as similar at least in effects to CBT (Gaudiano, 2011).

Person-centred therapy – changing low self-esteem

This approach is based on Carl Rogers' theory of the self, defined as 'the organized, consistent set of perceptions and beliefs about oneself' (Rogers, 1979). The self is composed of three components: (1) Self-worth: what we think about ourselves, developed in early childhood from the interaction of the child with the mother and father; (2) Self-image: how we see ourselves and (3) Ideal-self: the person who we would like to be which consists of our goals and ambitions in life. The self is considered to be in a dynamic state, with the potential for change in these three components.

This approach describes the self as influenced by the experiences a person has in their life and their interpretations of those experiences. Two primary sources are childhood experiences and evaluation by others. Self-actualisation occurs when a person's ideal self is congruent with their actual self. The closer our self-image and ideal-self are to each other, the more consistent or congruent we are and the higher our sense of self-worth. A person who has high self-worth, that is, has confidence and positive feelings about him or herself, faces challenges in life, accepts failure and unhappiness at times and is open with people.

Person-centred therapy, originated in the work of Carl Rogers, who believed that everyone is different and, therefore, everyone's view of their own world, and ability to manage it, should be trusted. Rogers believed that all of us have the power to find the best solutions for ourselves and make appropriate changes in our lives. Person-centred therapy was a movement away from the therapist's traditional role – as an expert – towards a process that allows clients to use their own understanding of their experiences as a platform for healing (Rogers, 1979). For a person to grow, they need an environment that provides them with genuineness (openness and self-disclosure), acceptance (being seen with unconditional positive regard) and empathy (being listened to and understood). Thus, the success of person-centred therapy relies on three conditions (Raskin & Rogers, 2005):

- Unconditional positive regard, to convey their feelings of understanding, trust and confidence that encourage clients to make their own decisions and choices.
- Empathetic understanding, which means therapists completely understand and accept their clients' thoughts and feelings.
- Congruence, which means therapists carry no air of authority or professional superiority but, instead, present a true and accessible self that clients can see is honest and transparent.

Person-centred therapy uses a non-authoritative approach that allows clients to take more of a lead in discussions so that, in the process, they will discover their own solutions. The therapist is there to encourage and support the client and to guide the therapeutic process without interrupting or interfering with the client's process of self-discovery. This approach is suited to individuals who want to gain more self-confidence, a stronger sense of identity, the ability to build healthy relationships and trust in their own decisions. In person-centred therapy, the client does most of the talking, the therapist does not interpret what is said but may restate what is said to fully understand the thoughts and feelings of the client in a non-judgemental way. This encourages the client to self-edit and clarify meaning. This may happen several times until the client decides that they have expressed exactly what they were thinking and feeling. This client-focused process facilitates self-discovery and self-acceptance, and provides a means towards healing and positive growth.

An evaluation of a primary care, person-centred counselling service utilised the Core Outcome Measure (CORE-OM) at referral and at the beginning and end of therapy on 697 individuals (Gibbard & Hanley, 2008) in order to assess effectiveness of the intervention. A pre–post therapy effect size over a five-year period was 1.2. This compared with a waitlist (between referral and pre-therapy) effect size of 0.24 for 382 individuals over a three-year period. The results indicate that person-centred counselling is effective with a modest effect size for clients with anxiety and depression (Gibbard & Hanley, 2008). It was also well supported by therapists (Daniel & Mcleod, 2006).

Attachment-based therapy – changing relating style

Attachment-based therapy is based on developing or rebuilding trusting relationships, and it centres on expressing emotion (Diamond, Shahar, Sabo, & Tsvieli, 2016). The therapist helps the client overcome negative early attachment issues by establishing a secure bond between the client and the therapist. The assumption being that they will then be better able to form healthy relationships with other people. Once the client–therapist relationship is established, the therapist can help the client communicate more openly and better explore and understand the connection between early attachment experiences and their current feelings and behaviours. However, many of the approaches are designed for children. For example, dyadic development psychotherapy (Beaumont, Jenkins, & Galpin, 2012) or ABC (Dozier, 2003) focuses on therapy with children, although foster parents are also included to improve parenting (Dozier, Albus, Fisher, & Sepulveda, 2002). These are outside the scope of this brief review.

Couples therapy and interpersonal therapy (IPT) – improving bonds with partners

Couples therapy has benefited from an attachment orientation similarly focused on relatedness (Johnson, 2003). The shared focus is also on the importance of developmental delays in the ability to form relationships, the lack of skills in communication or negotiation in partner relationships and misinterpretation, inferences or retaliation relating to the behavioural actions of the other. For example, those with an attachment style characterised by enmeshment/dependency can confuse caring behaviours and coercion tactics, and similarly, quid pro quo contracts are usually found in distressed, not happy couples (Bifulco & Thomas, 2012). The spouse/partner is viewed as the primary attachment figure for most adults and the main source of security and comfort. Proximity to an attachment figure usually reduces fear and feelings of helplessness. However, when this relationship is indifferent or conflictful, then the relationship becomes a turbulent rather than safe haven. The therapist seeks to improve communication skills and promote safe emotional engagement (Gottman & Levenson, 1992).

IPT treatment for patients with depression focuses on the past and present social roles and interpersonal interactions. During treatment, the therapist generally chooses one or two problem areas in the patient's current life to focus on. Examples of areas covered are disputes with friends, family or co-workers, grief and loss or role transitions, such as retirement or divorce.[3] IPT is usually based around four areas which are a mix of crises and vulnerabilities:

- **Unresolved grief:** In normal *bereavement*, the person usually begins to return to normal functioning within a few months. Unresolved grief is generally grief which is either delayed and experienced long after the loss or distorted grief, in which the person may not feel emotions, but instead experiences other symptoms.
- **Role disputes:** Role disputes occur when the patient and significant people in his/her life have different expectations about their relationship.
- **Role transitions:** Depression may occur during life transitions when a person's role changes and s/he doesn't know how to cope with the change.
- **Interpersonal deficits:** This may be an area of focus if the patient has had problems with forming and maintaining good quality relationships.

This approach has been well evaluated. A meta-analysis of randomised clinical trials of IPT efficacy for depression recovery was undertaken (de Mello, de Jesus Mari, Bacaltchuk, Verdeli, & Neugebauer, 2005). It found 13 studies which fulfilled inclusion criteria and four metaanalyses were performed. IPT was superior in efficacy to placebo in nine studies, had similar effects to medication and was significantly better than CBT. This suggests that IPT is an effective psychotherapy.

Mentalisation-based therapy (MBT) – seeing the mind of the other

An attachment approach combined with psychodynamic principles is utilised in Mentalisation-Based Therapy (Allen & Fonagy, 2006). Whilst often focused on adolescents, it also includes adult couples and families. It explores the limited psychological mindedness or 'capacity to interpret the behaviours of oneself and others in terms of mental states' of those who experienced childhood adversity. Poor mentalisation (reading the mind of others in relation to self) hinders emotional regulation and behavioural control. MBT promotes resilience by working on relational aspects in relatively brief (6–12 sessions) (Fearon et al., 2006). It also recognises the effects of stress and difficulty of mentalising when under stress and how this disrupts family relations (Bateman & Fonagy, 2000). The first evaluation of its use was with adolescents with a range of disorders including borderline personality disorder (Bo et al., 2017). This found that most of the 25 involved displayed improvement regarding borderline symptoms, depression, self-harm, peer-attachment, parent-attachment, mentalising and general psychopathology. Importantly, it also enhanced trust in peers and parents in combination with improved mentalising capacity. An eight-year follow-up of adults with personality disorder who had received 18 months of mentalisation-based treatment in hospital followed by 18 months of maintenance mentalising group therapy remain better than those receiving TAU (treatment as usual), but their general social function remains impaired (Bateman & Fonagy, 2008). Thus, this is an efficacious therapy but requiring some long-term delivery for personality disorder.

Discussion

This chapter sought to show how positive cognitive styles, support and positive life events contribute to wellbeing and form the mirror image to the vulnerability-provoking agent model of depression. The same needs model – Attachment, Security, Identity and Achievement – can be used to highlight positive frames of mind and positive experience which can add to these. This highlights that experiences can be positive and increase stability and enhance life, in addition to being negative and threatening. Most of us experience a mixture of these in our lives. Those resilient are able to glean more from such positive aspects.

Interventions which seek to make changes to vulnerability, in order to nurture more positive approaches to the world, have been outlined. There are fortunately a number of accepted and tested interventions for vulnerability to depression and anxiety. These seek to address negative aspects of thinking and feeling – whether through cognitive and behaviour change, acceptance or processing of childhood experience. The model developed throughout this book could aid therapists by pointing with greater precision to the types of vulnerability that might be present given the contextual information provided by the individual as well as providing possible measurement tools to assess these. Whilst the focus here has been on intensive interview measures, there are also questionnaires which can provide summary information – on attachment style, on self-esteem and on childhood experience. Being able to assess such factors may aid with identifying priorities in vulnerability; profiling and noting the numbers of such factors may also give an idea of level or 'dosages' of vulnerability risk.

Similarly, clinicians should recognise that positive events can emerge out of positive conditions but can also reflect the end of a negative situation. The likelihood of different types of positive event may be tied to various life stages with 'pure' positive events possibly more common in midlife (e.g. birth of a grandchild; cashing in a large pension; paying off a mortgage) and stabilising events more common in younger individuals (e.g. getting first permanent job). The likelihood of these events may also vary at different points in time; for instance, lower levels of home ownership along with lower pension pay-outs are more likely for younger people in the future. Many positive events are also related to socio-economic status and hence have the potential to heighten inequalities over the life-course due to the lower probability of some people experiencing them. This may have important implications for the relationship between positive events, disorder and opportunities for recovery in different groups in society.

Most treatments tend to occur for clients who are suffering psychological disorder, due to their vulnerability and life event crises co-occurring. However, for wider scale interventions, the potential for identifying vulnerable individuals prior to an episode (or indeed between episodes) could allow for preventative therapy to reduce sensitivity to future severe life events. This could alleviate pressure on health services as well as reduce distress to individuals if episodes of depression and anxiety could be averted through such early action. Indeed, given much vulnerability emanates from childhood experience, this could occur in late adolescence or early adulthood before long-term partner relationships and parenting were embarked upon. Such preventative work could be very beneficial.

Appraisal of positive events may be as critical for wellbeing as appraisal of negative events is for depression. Often, there is an assumption of over-sensitivity to events implied in vulnerability or robustness. Research is well attuned to the former but not to the latter. If some individuals cannot absorb positivity from events which are stabilising or enhancing, then creating these in intervention may help their social circumstances, but not affect their mood. So, therapy needs to not only amend negative ways of thinking but also inculcate positive ways of thinking and exploration of responsiveness to improve wellbeing. Thus, positive sense of self, of the world, the future and others (i.e. self-worth; meaningfulness, optimism and trust) needs to be the focus for those involved in promoting wellbeing. If these can exist as enduring states, perhaps in combination with improving the objective opportunities of all to experience some types of positive events. Then, positive events will serve to improve happier lives.

Notes

1 https://www.nhs.uk/conditions/cognitive-behavioural-therapy-cbt/
2 https://www.nhs.uk/conditions/cognitive-behavioural-therapy-cbt/
3 https://www.verywellmind.com/interpersonal-therapy-1067404

9 Conclusion

This book has sought to explicate in some detail the nature and characteristics of life events and the impact they can have on people's mental health and wellbeing. It has sought to argue that far from being standard categories of predictable change, life events are complex occurrences. They can be fraught with different forms of adverse experience and can change life plans, hopes and aspirations. They can also change close attachments, the course of life partnerships and plans for children. In this chapter, we will briefly summarise and draw out some further implications of the earlier discussions.

In order to understand severe life events in their rich complexity, we have outlined the classifications of loss, danger, humiliation and entrapment as features which run across the more prosaic event domain categories such as 'work' or 'housing'. We have explained in some detail how these are measured. Having such categorisations allows for a more theoretically meaningful analysis of such events. We have also put forward a model of how severe life events, due to these features, can damage our basic psychological needs of attachment, security, identity and achievement (ASIA) by interacting with personal vulnerability. On the positive side, we have shown secure attachment style to be associated with recovery from depression and to interact with positive events involving stabilising and enhancing characteristics in relating to high wellbeing. We have also showed the benefits of understanding life events in a time frame and in terms of sequences and their links to longer-term difficulties. This forms a context for the events with events later in the sequence taking a different meaning from the ones earlier as scenarios unfold. Such timing is also critical for research testing of when severe life events provoke episodes of emotional disorder or indeed are related to recovery from disorder.

We identified more than one type of vulnerability and sought to encapsulate proximal (recent) vulnerability in an attachment model, which also involved self-esteem to underpin the attachment, identity and achievement needs outlined in the ASIA model. This too is understood in terms of distal (childhood) vulnerability in terms of maltreatment, adversity and trauma, as a long-lasting legacy with implications for emotional disorder. This invokes damage to security and safety. Just as susceptibility to negative life events is shown in vulnerability factors, including negative self-esteem, problem relationships and insecure attachment style, so susceptibility to positive events can be shown in robustness features such as secure attachment and positive self-esteem. These have varied genetic and neurobiological underpinnings. For balance, we need to look at both negative and positive sides of life change and predisposing characteristics.

In terms of what can avert depression in the face of a severe life event, we have described crisis support at the time of the event as critical. This can inform intervention strategy both at the individual level but also for more universal services involved. A central element is the importance of confiding as a means of accessing effective support. Whilst this may sound simple, effective support actually requires a number of features being present. First, it requires the ability of an individual to communicate need when under stress. Second, it assumes the presence of a close and trusted figure who has provided emotional support on previous occasions. Third, for resilient support, it also requires alternative sources of confiding support should the first choice be unavailable. These sources may take the form of professional help. Both luck and timing may be involved in support availability – more than one support figure may be lost in a crisis (e.g. mother's untimely death deprives an individual of her support and that of a grieving sister, both circumstances outside her control). There is also a time constraint – the support figure is required to be available in what may be only a brief window of a few weeks to offer crucial support before depression takes hold. However, the presence of a support figure during a crisis can avert a depression even in vulnerable individuals. These are the types of research findings that can usefully inform interventions.

Positive events have also been shown to have a benign effect – both on recovery from clinical disorder and on wellbeing. However, not all individuals appear to be able to respond to positive events with the congruent emotions – negative cognitive biases seem to be able to override the benign changes implied. For some people, any change is a challenge; even positive change may undermine people's beliefs about whether they will cope, how the outside world will respond and whether they can really trust in the positive aspects of the change. For example, coping with a promotion, moving into better housing and starting a new relationship. For some, these will be fraught with fears of disappointment or failure. When individuals have positive cognitive sets, such events readily increase wellbeing. Therefore, therapy geared to increase positive mind sets will also aid with positive cascade effects when pleasurable events occur.

The factors encompassed in the vulnerability-provoking agent model presented in this book, and the different features and dimensions of life events point to the importance of thinking across a multi-dimensional model. We emphasised the socio-environmental approach in our introduction and have returned to it in different chapters in describing the wide range of crises that can occur to people to trigger disorder. We return here to consider how some of severe life events can be widespread in society, not only an issue of individual challenge. Some widespread events will have very practical ramifications impinging on individuals' sense of security – for example, having to leave home due to area flooding where the individual and others nearby are likely to need shelter, food and clothing. In such cases, community psychologists and social workers and the welfare system might be most appropriate to deal with the practical aspects of what has occurred. However, the loss of a home should not be underestimated as a psychological blow, and Maslow's model informs that the basic issues to do with security and safety need to be resolved before the psychological ones can effectively be tackled.

Similarly, some communal trauma events will create psychological and practical disturbance at all levels; for instance, war conflict will affect resources (e.g. disruption to food or water supplies), affect individuals (e.g. death of loved ones) and wider groups (e.g. divisions between religious groups) and geopolitical systems (visa and asylum issues). Events such as these need widescale resources and national policy input. Bearing in mind the different life arenas that can be impacted (e.g. through the ASIA model) and ascertaining which features have been activated (loss, danger, humiliation and entrapment) can have implications for morale, mental health and wellbeing not just at the individual level but at a community and national level.

A typical example would be the Covid-19 pandemic and considering how governments have managed it and its impact nationally and at local community and personal levels. Impacts are very varied. Thus, whilst some individuals have simply had their socialising curtailed in lockdown whilst they work from home, others have the potential for isolation, lack of care and support when ill, loss of close relatives to the virus where even the possibility of attending the funeral may be denied. Others will have lost income and work, whilst those in emergency services are working very long hours and putting their own health at risk. At this point, we do not know how long this will last, but it is clear that all levels of society are involved, and the impacts on individuals are likely to be high. This has implications for community psychology approaches in addition to the predictive expertise of epidemiologists and public health experts. There are many who see a second major wave of ill health as psychological.

Community psychology is fundamentally concerned with the relationship between social systems and individual wellbeing in the community context. Influenced by the socio-ecological model, it integrates social, cultural, economic, political, environmental and international influences to promote positive change, health and empowerment at individual and systemic levels (Rappaport & Seidman, 2000). It promotes mental health and community wellbeing and seeks to better understand the multiple influences of the social environment on health and wellbeing. The focus is not only on individual vulnerability but also on multiple levels of analysis from individuals and groups to specific organisations and, finally, to whole communities. In this, psychological disorder is located as a product of community conditions.

Given community psychologists are more likely to see threats to mental health in the social environment, or in a lack of fit between individuals and their environment, this leads to advocating social rather than individual change. They also have a focus on health rather than on illness and on enhancing individual and community competencies. There is therefore an interest in preventative work to tackle problems at an early stage, rather than waiting for them to become serious and debilitating. When effective, this can help the relatively powerless take control over their environment and their lives by providing and evaluating an array of programs and policies which help people manage the stressful aspects of community and organisational environments. For example, in the aftermath of the Grenfell Tower fire in London, a community response was very much mobilised. Individual work came later looking at aspects of trauma and how the crisis impacted on the individuals involved considering their personal vulnerability profile.

Public policy and population mental health and wellbeing

Having illustrated in earlier chapters, some of the therapies and interventions available for tackling vulnerability and severe life events which lead to clinical disorder, we now briefly outline current public policy on mental health in the UK. This also includes actions to combat life events which occur on a community-wide scale. Public policy on mental health in England has a five-year plan[1] to develop three key overlapping areas of public mental health across the life course:

- mental health promotion
- prevention of mental health problems and suicide prevention
- improving lives, supporting recovery and inclusion of people living with mental health problems.

On the world stage, at an international level, the World Health Organisation similarly lists the need for coordinated planning.[2] Here, a focus is placed on mental health at a population level to consider frameworks required to have far reaching effects. This requires coordination of essential services around delivery to those in need, clear definitions of targets/outcomes and detailing the responsibilities of those involved:

> A mental health plan is a pre-formulated detailed scheme to implement the vision and objectives defined in the policy. A plan should include the concrete strategies and activities that will be implemented to tackle mental disorders and associated disability, as well as specifying the targets to be achieved by the government. It should also clarify the roles of the different stakeholders in implementing the activities of the mental health plan. https://www.who.int/mental_health/policy/services/en/

At the time of writing, the global pandemic of Covid-19 virus is affecting physical and mental health on an international scale (Brooks et al., 2020). At this point, we do not know how long it will last or how it well end. It is currently leading to high-mortality rates in those older and with pre-existing health conditions and those in certain ethnic groups as well as men who contract it. It is leading to huge social disruption with people self-isolating and businesses closing. At point of lockdown, there was virtual economic shutdown with the government expending billions. This has led to individual experience of severe life events and even trauma experiences on a population basis. The recommended social distancing or shielding, in terms of keeping distance from those close if not in the household, is at odds with the usual recommendations of psychologists to increase opportunities for close communication and confiding when managing crises. This is a challenge not just for physical health services but also for those involved in mental health as the impacts on economic factors, loss of those close and lack of geographical mobility start to take a toll. Understanding within this context the nature of crises in the form of life events, and what makes these unpleasant and threatening and how individuals can be susceptible or resilient to their impacts is important psychoeducational knowledge in preserving the mental health and wellbeing of individuals.

Conclusion

The book has sought to bring to the fore existing knowledge about life events to explain what they are and what impacts they can have on individual emotional disorder, on mental health more generally and on wellbeing. The origins of negative life events are conceptualised in a socio-ecological framework with an emphasis on social deprivation and inequality. The extent of the impact of such events on individuals leads back to early life experiences and the psychological and neurobiological vulnerability factors than can occur. Much of what is covered in this book was established by the end of the 20th century – the newer elements are around digitally based methods and treatments and the biological bases for vulnerability – as well as the synthesis of the varied study findings. However, much of what we know of the importance of life events in terms of the depth and nuance of the approach seems to have been overlooked by the current generation of researchers and clinical practitioners. This is in part due to an over-simplification of measures adopted for life events research which has reduced them to proscribed checklists but also the intense focus on both cognitive and genetic factors has perhaps de-emphasised the very large contribution of such negative changes from the social environment. We hope that we have readdressed this balance and that this revisiting of life events will be used to aid further research and practice.

We should not underestimate the power of events – in the words of Robert Penn Warren in his novel 'All the Kings Men' writing about the 1930s American south and a split society racially (Warren, 2007):

> After a great blow, or crisis, after the first shock and then after the nerves have stopped screaming and twitching, you settle down to the new condition of things and feel that all possibility of change has been used up. You adjust yourself, and are sure that the new equilibrium is for eternity... But if anything is certain it is that no story is ever over, for the story which we

think is over is only a chapter in a story which will not be over, and it isn't the game that is over, it is just an inning, and that game has a lot more than nine innings. When the game stops it will be called on account of darkness. But it is a long day.

—Robert Penn Warren, All the King's Men (1946)

Notes

1 https://www.gov.uk/government/collections/public-mental-health
2 https://www.who.int/mental_health/policy/services/en/

References

Abdul Kadir, N.B., & Bifulco, A. (2011). Vulnerability, life events and depression among Moslem Malaysian women – comparing those married and those divorced or separated. *Social Psychiatry & Psychiatric Epidemiology, 46*, 855–862. doi: 10.1007/s00127-010-0249-4

Abela, J.R. (2002). Depressive mood reactions to failure in the achievement domain: A test of the integration of the hopelessness and self-esteem theories of depression. *Cognitive Therapy and Research, 26*(4), 531–552.

Ainsworth, M.D.S., Blehar, M., Aters, E., & Wall, S. (1978). *Patterns of attachment: A psychological study of the strange situation.* Hillsdale, NJ: Lawrence, Erlbaum.

Allen, J.G., & Fonagy, P. (2006). *Handbook of mentalization treatment.* Chichester: John Wiley and Sons.

Alloy, L.B., Abramson, L.Y., Safford, S.M., & Gibb, B.E. (2006). The cognitive vulnerability to depression (CVD) project: Current findings and future directions. In Alloy, L.B., Riskind, J.H. (Eds.), *Cognitive vulnerability to emotional disorders* (pp. 43–72): London: Routledge.

Anastasia, A., Deinhardt, K., Chao, M.V., Will, N.E., Irmady, K., Lee, F.S., … Bracken, C. (2013). Val66Met polymorphism of BDNF alters prodomain structure to induce neuronal growth cone retraction. *Nature Communications, 4*(1), 2490. doi: 10.1038/ncomms3490

Anders, S.L., Frazier, P.A., & Frankfurt, S.B. (2011). Variations in Criterion A and PTSD rates in a community sample of women. *Journal of Anxiety Disorders, 25*(2), 176–184. doi: 10.1016/j.janxdis.2010.08.018

Anderson, B., Wethington, E., & Kamarck, T.W. (2010). Interview assessment of stressor exposure. In R.J. Contrada, & A. Baum (Eds.), *The handbook of stress science: Biology, psychology, and health.* Berlin: Springer.

Andersson, G., & Cuijpers, P. (2008). Pros and cons of online cognitive–behavioural therapy. *The British Journal of Psychiatry, 193*(4), 270–271.

Andersson, G., Rozental, A., Shafran, R., & Carlbring, P. (2018). Long-term effects of internet-supported cognitive behaviour therapy. *Expert Review of Neurotherapeutics, 18*(1), 21–28.

Andersson, G., Titov, N., Dear, B.F., Rozental, A., & Carlbring, P. (2019). Internet-delivered psychological treatments: From innovation to implementation. *World Psychiatry, 18*(1), 20–28.

Andersson, G., Topooco, N., Havik, O., & Nordgreen, T. (2016). Internet-supported versus face-to-face cognitive behavior therapy for depression. *Expert Review of Neurotherapeutics, 16*(1), 55–60.

Andrews, B., Brewin, C.R., Rose, S., & Kirk, M. (2000). Predicting PTSD symptoms in victims of violent crime: The role of shame, anger, and childhood abuse. *Journal of Abnormal Psychology, 109*(1), 69. doi: 10.1037/0021–843X.109.1.69

Andrews, B., & Brown, G.W. (1988). Marital violence in the community: A biographical approach. *British Journal of Psychiatry, 153*, 305–312.

APA. (2013). *Diagnostic and statistical manual of mental disorders (DSM-5®).* Arlington, VA: American Psychiatric Association.

Asselmann, E., Wittchen, H., Lieb, R., Hofler M, & Beesdo-Baum, K. (2015). Danger and loss events and the incidence of anxiety and depressive disorders: A prospective-longitudinal community study of adolescents and young adults. *Psychological Medicine, 45*, 153–163. doi: 10.1017/S0033291714001160

Atwoli, L., Stein, D.J., Koenen, K.C., & McLaughlin, K.A. (2015). Epidemiology of post-traumatic stress disorder: Prevalence, correlates and consequences. *Current Opinion in Psychiatry, 28*(4), 307–311. doi: 10.1097/yco.0000000000 000167

Bakermans-Kranenburg, M.J., & IJzendoorn, M.H.v. (2007). Research review: Genetic vulnerability or differential susceptibility in child development: The case of attachment. *Journal of Child Psychology and Psychiatry, 48*(12), 1160–1173.

Bakermans-Kranenburg, M.J., & van Ijzendoorn, M.H. (2006). Gene-environment interaction of the dopamine D4 receptor (DRD4) and observed maternal insensitivity predicting externalizing behavior in preschoolers. *Developmental Psychobiology, 48*, 406–409.

Baldwin, M.W., & Sinclair, L. (1996). Self-esteem and "if... then" contingencies of interpersonal acceptance. *Journal of Personality and Social Psychology, 71*(6), 1130.

Barber, B.K., McNeely, C., Olsen, J.A., Belli, R.F., & Doty, S.B. (2016). Long-term exposure to political violence: The particular injury of persistent humiliation. *Social Science & Medicine, 156*, 154–166.

Barnes, J., Belsky, J., Broomfield, K.A., Dave, S., Frost, M., Melhuish, E., & Team, T.N.E.o.S.S.R. (2005). Disadvantaged but different: Variation among deprived communities in relation to child and family well-being. *Journal of Child Psychology and Psychiatry, 46*(9), 952–962.

Barnes, J., & Stein, A. (2000). Effects of parental psychiatric and physical illness on child development. In M. Gelder, J.J. Lopez-Ibor, & N. Andreasen (Eds.), *New Oxford textbook of psychiatry.* Oxford: Oxford University Press.

Bartholomew, K., & Horowitz, L.M. (1991). Attachment styles among young adults: A test of a four-category model. *Journal of Personality and Social Psychology, 61*(2), 226–244.

Bateman, A., & Fonagy, P. (2000). Effectiveness of psychotherapeutic treatment of personality disorder. *British Journal of Psychiatry, 177*, 138–143.

Bateman, A., & Fonagy, P. (2008). 8-year follow-up of patients treated for borderline personality disorder: Mentalization-based treatment versus treatment as usual. *American Journal of Psychiatry, 165*(5), 631–638.

Beaumont, E., Jenkins, P., & Galpin, A. (2012). 'Being kinder to myself': A prospective comparative study, exploring post-trauma therapy outcome measures, for two groups of clients, receiving either cognitive behaviour therapy or cognitive behaviour therapy and compassionate mind training. *Counselling Psychology Review, 27*(1), 31–43.

Bebbington, P.E., Dean, C., Der, G., Hurry, J., & et al. (1991). Gender, parity and the prevalence of minor affective disorder. *British Journal of Psychiatry, 158*, 40–45.

Beck, A.T. (1967). *Depression: clinical, experimental and theoretical perspectives.* New York: Hoeber.

Beck, A.T., & Bredemeier, K. (2016). A unified model of depression: Integrating clinical, cognitive, biological, and evolutionary perspectives. *Clinical Psychological Science, 4*(4), 596–619. doi: 10.1177/2167702616628523

Belli, R.F., Shay, W.L., & Stafford, F.P. (2001). Event history calendars and question list surveys: A direct comparison of interviewing methods. *Public Opinion Quarterly, 65*(1), 45–74.

Belsky, J., Bakermans-Kranenburg, M.J., & Van IJzendoorn, M.H. (2007). For better and for worse: Differential susceptibility to environmental influences. *Current Directions in Psychological Science, 16*(6), 300–304.

Belsky, J., Jonassaint, C., Pluess, M., Stanton, M., Brummett, B., & Williams, R. (2009). Vulnerability genes or plasticity genes? *Molecular Psychiatry, 14*(8), 746–754.

Belsky, J., & Nezworski, T. (1987). *Clinical implications of attachment.* London: Lawrence Erlbaum Associates.

Belsky, J., & Pluess, M. (2009). Beyond diathesis stress: Differential susceptibility to environmental influences. *Psychological Bulletin, 135*(6), 885.

Belsky, J., & Van Ijzendoorn, M. (2015). What works for whom? Genetic moderation of intervention efficacy. *Development and Psychopathology, 27*(1), 1–6. doi: 10.1017/S0954579414001254

Bennett, B., Repacholi, M., & Carr, Z. (2006). *Health effects of the Chernobyl accident and special health care programmes: Report of the UN Chernobyl forum health expert group.* Retrieved from Geneva. https://www.who.int/ionizing_radiation/chernobyl/WHO%20Report%20on%20Chernobyl%20Health%20Effects%20July%202006.pdf

Berry, K., Barrowclough, C., & Wearden, A. (2007). A review of the role of adult attachment style in psychosis: Unexplored issues and questions for further research. *Clinical Psychology Review, 27*, 458.

Bifulco, A., Bernazzani, O., Moran, P.M., & Ball, C. (2000). Lifetime stressors and recurrent depression: Preliminary findings of the adult life phase interview (ALPHI). *Social Psychiatry and Psychiatric Epidemiology, 35*, 264–275. doi: 10.1007/s001270050238

Bifulco, A., & Brown, G.W. (1996). Cognitive coping response to crises and onset of depression. *Social Psychiatry and Psychiatric Epidemiology, 31*, 163–172.

Bifulco, A., Brown, G.W., & Adler, Z. (1991). Early sexual abuse and clinical depression in adult life. *British Journal of Psychiatry, 159*, 115–122. doi: 10.1192/bjp.159.1.115

Bifulco, A., Brown, G.W., & Harris, T.O. (1987). Childhood loss of parent, lack of adequate parental care and adult depression: A replication. *Journal of Affective Disorders, 12*, 115–128.

Bifulco, A., Brown, G.W., & Harris, T.O. (1994). Childhood experience of care and abuse (CECA): A retrospective interview measure. *Journal of Child Psychology and Psychiatry, 35*, 1419–1435. doi: 10.1111/j.1469–7610.1994.tb01284.x

Bifulco, A., Brown, G.W., Lillie, A., & Jarvis, J. (1997). Memories of childhood neglect and abuse: Corroboration in a series of sisters. *Journal of Child Psychology and Psychiatry, 38*, 365–374. doi: 10.1111/j.1469–7610.1997.tb01520.x

Bifulco, A., Brown, G.W., Moran, P., Ball, C., & Campbell, C. (1998). Predicting depression in women: The role of past and present vulnerability. *Psychological Medicine, 28*(1), 39–50.

Bifulco, A., Damiani, R., Jacobs, C., & Spence, R. (2019). Partner violence in women – associations with major depression, attachment style and childhood maltreatment. *Maltrattamento e abuso all'infanzia, 21*, 13–28.

Bifulco, A., Harris, T., & Brown, G.W. (1992). Mourning or early inadequate care? Reexamining the relationship of maternal loss in childhood with adult depression and anxiety. *Development and Psychopathology, 4*, 433–449.

Bifulco, A., Jacobs, C., Oskis, A., Cavana F., & Spence, R. (2019). Lifetime trauma, adversity and emotional disorder in older age women. *Maltrattamento e abuso all'infanzia, 21*, 29–43.

Bifulco, A., Kagan, L., Spence, R., Nunn, S., Bailey-Rodriquez, D., Hosang, G.M., … Fisher, H.L. (2019). Characteristics of severe life events, attachment style and depression – Using an online approach. *The British Journal of Clinical Psychology*, 8(4), 427–439. doi: 10.1111/bjc.1221

Bifulco, A., Kwon, J.H., Moran, P.M., Jacobs, C., Bunn, A., & Beer, N. (2006). Adult attachment style as mediator between childhood neglect/abuse and adult depression and anxiety. *Social Psychiatry & Psychiatric Epidemiology*, 41(10), 796–805. doi: 10.1007/s00127-006-0101-z

Bifulco, A., Mahon, J., Kwon, J.-H., Moran, P., & Jacobs, C. (2003). The vulnerable attachment style questionnaire (VASQ): An interview-derived measure of attachment styles that predict depressive disorder. *Psychological Medicine*, 33, 1099–1110. doi: 10.1017/S0033291703008237

Bifulco, A., & Moran, P. (1998). *Wednesday's child: Research into women's experience of neglect and abuse in childhood and adult depression.* London, New York: Routledge.

Bifulco, A., Moran, P., Baines, R., Bunn, A., & Stanford, K. (2003). Exploring psychological abuse in childhood: II. Association with other abuse and adult clinical depression. *Bulletin of the Menninger Clinic*, 66, 241–258. doi: 10.1521/bumc.66.3.241.23366

Bifulco, A., Moran, P.M., Ball, C., & Bernazzani, O. (2002). Adult attachment style. I: Its relationship to clinical depression. *Social Psychiatry & Psychiatric Epidemiology*, 37, 50–59. doi: 10.1007/s127-002-8215-0

Bifulco, A., Moran, P.M., Ball, C., Jacobs, C., Baines, R., Bunn, A., & Cavagin, J. (2002). Childhood adversity, parental vulnerability and disorder: Examining intergenerational transmission of risk. *Journal of Child Psychology and Psychiatry*, 43, 1075–1086.

Bifulco, A., Moran, P.M., Ball, C., & Lillie, A. (2002). Adult attachment style. II: Its relationship to psychosocial depressive-vulnerability. *Social Psychiatry & Psychiatric Epidemiology*, 37, 60–67. doi: 10.1007/s127-002-8216-x

Bifulco, A., & Schimmenti, A. (2019). Assessing child abuse: "We need to talk!". *Child Abuse & Neglect*, 98, 104236. doi: 10.1016/j.chiabu.2019.104236

Bifulco, A., Schimmenti, A., Moran, P., Jacobs, C., Bunn, A., & Rusu, A.C. (2014). Problem parental care and teenage deliberate self-harm in young community adults. *Bulletin of the Menninger Clinic*, 78(2), 95–114. doi: 10.1521/bumc.2014.78.2.95

Bifulco, A., Spence, R., Nunn, S., Kagan, L., Rodriguez, D., Hosang G.M., … Fisher, H.L. (2019). The computerised life events and assessment record (CLEAR) online measure of life events: Reliability, validity and association with depression. *JMIR Mental Health*, 6(1), e10675. doi: 10.2196/10675

Bifulco, A., & Thomas, G. (2012). *Understanding adult attachment in family relationships: Research, assessment and intervention.* London: Routledge.

Binnie, J. (2015). Do you want therapy with that? A critical account of working within IAPT. *Mental Health Review Journal*, 20 (2), 79–83.

Binnie, J. (2018). Medical approaches to suffering are limited, so why critique improving access to psychological therapies from the same ideology. *Journal of Health Psychology*, 23(9), 1159–1162.

Bleys, D., Luyten, P., Soenens, B., & Claes, S. (2018). Gene-environment interactions between stress and 5-HTTLPR in depression: A meta-analytic update. *Journal of Affective Disorders*, 226, 339–345. doi: 10.1016/j.jad.2017.09.050

Bo, S., Sharp, C., Beck, E., Pedersen, J., Gondan, M., & Simonsen, E. (2017). First empirical evaluation of outcomes for mentalization-based group therapy for adolescents with BPD. *Personality Disorders: Theory, Research, and Treatment*, 8(4), 396.

Bodkin, J.A., Pope, H.G., Detke, M.J., & Hudson, J.I. (2007). Is PTSD caused by traumatic stress? *Journal of Anxiety Disorders*, 21(2), 176–182. doi: 10.1016/j.janxdis.2006.09.004

Boscarino, J.A. (2004). Posttraumatic stress disorder and physical illness: Results from clinical and epidemiologic studies. *Annals of the New York Academy of Sciences, 1032,* 141–153. doi: 10.1196/annals.1314.011

Boscarino, J.A., & Adams, R.E. (2009). PTSD onset and course following the World Trade Center disaster: Findings and implications for future research. *Social Psychiatry and Psychiatric Epidemiology, 44*(10), 887–898. doi: 10.1007/s00127-009-0011-y

Bottonari, K.A., Safren, S.A., McQuaid, J.R., Hsiao, C.-B., & Roberts, J.E. (2010). A longitudinal investigation of the impact of life stress on HIV treatment adherence. *Journal of Behavioral Medicine, 33*(6), 486–495.

Bowlby, J. (1951). *Maternal care and mental health WHO, Geneva.* Retrieved from https://pages.uoregon.edu/eherman/teaching/texts/Bowlby%20Maternal%20Care%20and%20Mental%20Health.pdf

Bowlby, J. (1977). Aetiology and psychopathology in the light of attachment theory. *British Journal of Psychiatry, 130,* 201–210.

Bowlby, J. (1979). *The making and breaking of affectional bonds.* London: Routledge.

Bowlby, J. (1980). *Attachment and loss: vol 3. Loss; sadness and depression.* New York: Basic Books.

Bowlby, J. (1988). *A secure base: Clinical application of attachment theory.* London: Routledge.

Brewin, C.R. (2001). Cognitive and emotional reactions to traumatic events: Implications for short-term intervention. *Advances in Mind-Body Medicine, 17*(3), 163–168. https://psycnet.apa.org/record/2001-18075-001

Brewin, C.R. (2014). Episodic memory, perceptual memory, and their interaction: Foundations for a theory of posttraumatic stress disorder. *Psychological Bulletin, 140*(1), 69. doi: 10.1037/a0033722

Brewin, C.R., Andrews, B., & Valentine, J.D. (2000). Meta-analysis of risk factors for posttraumatic stress disorder in trauma-exposed adults. *Journal of Consulting and Clinical Psychology, 68*(5), 748–766. doi: 10.1037/0022-006X.68.5.748

Broadhead, J., & Abas, M. (1998). Life events, difficulties and depression among women in an urban setting in Zimbabwe. *Psychological Medicine, 28*(1). doi: 10.1017/S0033291797005618

Bronfenbrenner, U. (1995). Developmental ecology through space and time: A future perspective. In P. Moen & G.H. Elder, Jr. (Eds.), *Examining lives in context: Perspectives on the ecology of human development* (pp. 619–647). Washington, DC: American Psychological Association.

Brooker, C., & Brabban, A. (2004). *Measured success: A scoping review of evaluated psychosocial interventions training for work with people with serious mental health problems.* Retrieved from http://eprints.lincoln.ac.uk/id/eprint/742/

Brooks, S.K., Webster, R.K., Smith, L.E., Woodland, L., Wessely, S., Greenberg, N., & Rubin, G.J. (2020). The psychological impact of quarantine and how to reduce it: Rapid review of the evidence. *The Lancet, 395,* 912–920.

Brown, G.W. (1972). Life events and psychiatric illness: Some thoughts on methodology and causality. *Journal of Psychosomatic Research, 1981; 25(5): 461 473, 16,* 311–320.

Brown, G.W. (1993). Life events and affective disorder: Replications and limitations. *Psychosomatic Medicine, 55,* 248–259.

Brown, G.W., Adler, Z., & Bifulco, A. (1988). Life events, difficulties and recovery from chronic depression. *British Journal of Psychiatry, 152,* 487–498.

Brown, G.W., Andrews, B., Bifulco, A., & Veiel, H.O. (1990). Self esteem and depression: I. Measurement issues and prediction of onset. *Social Psychiatry and Psychiatric Epidemiology, 25,* 200–209. doi: 10.1007/BF00788643

Brown, G.W., Andrews, B., Harris, T., Adler, Z., & Bridge, L. (1986). Social support, self-esteem and depression. *Psychological Medicine, 16*(4), 813–831.

Brown, G.W., Ban, M., Craig, T.K., Harris, T.O., Herbert, J., & Uher, R. (2013). Serotonin transporter length polymorphism, childhood maltreatment, and chronic depression: A specific gene–environment interaction. *Depression and Anxiety, 30*(1), 5–13.

Brown, G.W., Bifulco, A., & Andrews, B. (1990a). Self-esteem and depression: III. Aetiological issues. *Social Psychiatry and Psychiatric Epidemiology, 25*, 235–243.

Brown, G.W., Bifulco, A., & Andrews, B. (1990b). Self-esteem and depression: IV. Effect on course and recovery. *Social Psychiatry and Psychiatric Epidemiology, 25*, 244–249.

Brown, G.W., Bifulco, A., & Harris, T. (1987). Life events, vulnerability and onset of depression: Some refinements. *British Journal of Psychiatry, 150*, 30–42. doi: 10.1192/bjp.150.1.30

Brown, G.W., Bifulco, A., Veil, H.O., & Andrews, B. (1990). Self-esteem and depression: II. Social correlates of self-esteem. *Social Psychiatry and Psychiatric Epidemiology, 25*, 225–234.

Brown, G.W., Craig, T.K.J., Harris, T.O., Herbert, J., Hodgson, K., Tansey, K.E., & Rudolf, U. (2013). Functional polymorphism in the brain-derived neurotrophic factor gene interacts with stressful life events but not childhood maltreatment in the etiology of depression. *Depression and Anxiety, 0*, 1–9. doi: 10.1002/da.22221

Brown, G.W., & Harris, T.O. (1978). *Social origins of depression: A study of psychiatric disorder in women.* London, New York: Tavistock.

Brown, G.W., & Harris, T.O. (1989). *Life events and illness.* New York: Guillford Press.

Brown, G.W., Harris, T.O., & Hepworth, C. (1995). Loss, humiliation and entrapment among women developing depression: A patient and non-patient comparison. *Psychological Medicine, 25*, 7–21. doi: 10.1017/S003329170002804X

Brown, G.W., Lemyre, L., & Bifulco, A. (1992). Social factors and recovery from anxiety and depressive disorders: A test of specificity. *British Journal of Psychiatry, 161*, 44–54. doi: 10.1192/bjp.161.1.44

Brown, G.W., Sklair, F., Harris, T.O., & Birley, J.L.T. (1973). Life events and psychiatric disorders, I: Some methodological issues. *Psychological Medicine, 3*, 74–87.

Brown, J.D., Dutton, K.A., & Cook, K.E. (2001). From the top down: Self-esteem and self-evaluation. *Cognition and Emotion, 15*(5), 615–631.

Brown, J.D., & McGill, K.L. (1989). The cost of good fortune: When positive life events produce negative health consequences. *Journal of Personality and Social Psychology, 57*(6), 1103.

Brown, M., Glendenning, A.C., Hoon, A.E., & John, A. (2016). Effectiveness of web-delivered acceptance and commitment therapy in relation to mental health and well-being: A systematic review and meta-analysis. *Journal of Medical Internet Research, 18*(8), e221.

Brugha, T., Bebbington, P., Tennant, C., & Hurry, J. (Feb 1985). The list of threatening experiences: A subset of 12 life event categories with considerable long-term contextual threat. *Psychological Medicine: A Journal of Research in Psychiatry and the Allied Sciences, 15*(1), 189–194.

Brugha, T.S., & Cragg, D. (1990). The list of threatening experiences: The reliability and validity of a brief life events questionaire. *Acta Psyciatrica Scandinavia, 82*, 77–81. doi: 10.1111/j.1600-0447.1990.tb01360.x

Buchanan, T. (2007). Personality testing on the Internet. In A.N. Joinson, K. McKenna, T. Postmes, & U.-D. Reips (Eds.), *Oxford handbook of Internet psychology*, 447–460. Oxford: Oxford University Press.

Buchanan, T., Johnson, J.A., & Goldberg, L.R. (2005). Implementing a five-factor personality inventory for use on the internet. *European Journal of Psychological Assessment, 21*(2), 115–127.

Buhrmester, M., Kwang, T., & Gosling, S.D. (2016). Amazon's mechanical turk: A new source of inexpensive, yet high-quality data? In A.E. Kazdin (Ed.), *Methodological issues and strategies in clinical research* (pp. 133–139). American Psychological Association. doi: 10.1037/14805-009

Cabizuca, M., Marques-Portella, C., Mendlowicz, M.V., Coutinho, E.S., & Figueira, I. (2009). Posttraumatic stress disorder in parents of children with chronic illnesses: A meta-analysis. *Health Psychology, 28*(3), 379. doi: 10.1037/a0014512

Carey, P.D., Stein, D.J., Zungu-Dirwayi, N., & Seedat, S. (2003). Trauma and post-traumatic stress disorder in an urban Xhosa primary care population: Prevalence, comorbidity, and service use patterns. *The Journal of Nervous and Mental Disease, 191*(4), 230–236. doi: 10.1097/01.NMD.0000061143.66146.A8

Carlbring, P., Andersson, G., Cuijpers, P., Riper, H., & Hedman-Lagerlöf, E. (2018). Internet-based vs. face-to-face cognitive behavior therapy for psychiatric and somatic disorders: An updated systematic review and meta-analysis. *Cognitive Behaviour Therapy, 47*(1), 1–18.

Carleton, R.N., Peluso, D.L., Collimore, K.C., & Asmundson, G.J.G. (2011). Social anxiety and posttraumatic stress symptoms: The impact of distressing social events. *Journal of Anxiety Disorders, 25*(1), 49–57. doi: 10.1016/j.janxdis.2010.08.002

Carlson, E.B., Smith, S.R., & Dalenberg, C.J. (2013). Can sudden, severe emotional loss be a traumatic stressor? *Journal of Trauma & Dissociation, 14*(5), 519–528. doi: 10.1080/15299732.2013.773475

Carlson, M., & Earls, F. (1997). Psychological and neuroendocrinological sequelae of early social deprivation in institutionalized children in Romania. *The Integrative Neurobiology of Affiliation, 807*(1), 419–428.

Carmassi, C., Dell'Osso, L., Manni, C., Candini, V., Dagani, J., Iozzino, L., … de Girolamo, G. (2014). Frequency of trauma exposure and post-traumatic stress disorder in Italy: Analysis from the World mental health survey initiative. *Journal of Psychiatric Research, 59*, 77–84. doi: 10.1016/j.jpsychires.2014.09.006

Caspi, A., Hariri, A., Holmes, A., Uher, R., & Moffitt, T.E. (2010). Genetic sensitivity to the environment: The case of serotonin transporter gene (5-HTTT) and its implications for studying complex diseases and traits. *American Journal of Psychiatry, 167*(5), 509–527.

Caspi, A., Sugden, K., Moffitt, T.E., Taylor, A., Craig, I.W., Harrington, H., … Braithwaite, A. (2003). Influence of life stress on depression: Moderation by a polymorphism in the 5-HTT gene. *Science, 301*(5631), 386–389.

Cassidy, J., & Shaver, P.R. (Eds.). (1999). *Handbook of attachment: Theory, research, and clinical applications*. New York: The Guilford Press.

Chandrashekar, P. (2018). Do mental health mobile apps work: Evidence and recommendations for designing high-efficacy mental health mobile apps. *Mhealth, 4*, 6 doi: 10.21037/mhealth.2018.03.02

Chaudhry, N., Husain, N., Tomenson, B., & Creed, F. (2012). A prospective study of social difficulties, acculturation and persistent depression in Pakistani women living in the UK. *Psychological Medicine, 42*(6), 1217–1226.

Choi, H., & Marks, N.F. (2008). Marital conflict, depressive symptoms, and functional impairment. *Journal of Marriage and Family, 70*(2), 377–390.

Chu, B.C., & Harrison, T.L. (2007). Disorder-specific effects of CBT for anxious and depressed youth: A meta-analysis of candidate mediators of change. *Clinical Child and Family Psychology Review, 10*(4), 352–372.

Chuah, S.C., Drasgow, F., & Roberts, B.W. (2006). Personality assessment: Does the medium matter? No. *Journal of Research in Personality, 40*(4), 359–376.

Cicchetti, D. (1996). Child maltreatment: Implications for developmental theory and research. *Human Development, 39*(1), 18–39.

Cicchetti, D., & Rogosch, F.A. (2001). The impact of child maltreatment and psychopathology on neuroendocrine functioning. *Development and Psychopathology, 13*(4), 783–804.

Ciechanowski, P., Katon, W., & Russo, J. (2005). The association of depression and perceptions of interpersonal relationships in patients with diabetes. *Journal of Psychosomatic Research, 58*, 139–144.

Ciechanowski, P.S., Katon, W.J., Russo, J., & Dwight-Johnson, M. (2002). Association of attachment style to lifetime medically unexplained symptoms in patients with hepatitis C. *Psychosomatics, 43*, 206.

Clark, D.M. (2018). Realizing the mass public benefit of evidence-based psychological therapies: The IAPT program. *Annual Review of Clinical Psychology, 14*, 159–183.

Cohen, J.A., & Mannarino, A.P. (2008). Trauma-focused cognitive behavioural therapy for children and parents. *Child and Adolescent Mental Health, 13*(4), 158–162.

Collazzoni, A., Capanna, C., Bustini, M., Marucci, C., Prescenzo, S., Ragusa, M., & et al. (2015). A comparison of humiliation measurement in a depressive versus nonclinical sample: A possible clinical utility. *Journal of Clinical Psychology, 71*, 1218–1224. doi: 10.1002/jclp.22212

Conger, R.D., & Elder, G.H. (1994). *Families in troubled times: Adapting to change in rural America*. New York: Aldine.

Conrad-Hiebner, A., & Scanlon, E. (2015). The economic conditions of child physical abuse: A call for a national research, policy, and practice agenda. *Families in Society: The Journal of Contemporary Social Services, 96*, 59–66. doi: 10.1606/1044-3894.2015.96.8

Contractor, A.A., Durham, T.A., Brennan, J.A., Armour, C., Wutrick, H.R., Frueh, B.C., & Elhai, J.D. (2014). DSM-5 PTSD's symptom dimensions and relations with major depression's symptom dimensions in a primary care sample. *Psychiatry Research, 215*(1), 146–153. doi: 10.1016/j.psychres.2013.10.015

Cowen, P.J. (2002). Cortisol, serotonin and depression: all stressed out? *British Journal of Psychiatry, 180*, 99–100.

Cowen, P.J., & Browning, M. (2015). What has serotonin to do with depression? *World Psychiatry: Official Journal of the World Psychiatric Association (WPA), 14*(2), 158–160. doi: 10.1002/wps.20229

Cozolino, L.J. (2005). The impact of trauma on the brain. *Psychotherapy in Australia, 11*(3), 22.

Cozzarelli, C., Karafa, J.A., Collins, N.L., & Tagler, M.J. (2003). Stability and change in adult attachment styles: Associations with personal vulnerabilities, life events, and global construals of self and others. *Journal of Social and Clinical Psychology, 22*, 315–346.

Craig, T.K.J., & Brown, G.W. (1994). Goal frustration and life events in the aetiology of painful gastrointestinal disorder. *Journal of Psychosomatic Research, 28*(5), 411–421.

Culverhouse, R.C., Saccone, N.L., Horton, A.C., Ma, Y., Anstey, K.J., Banaschewski, T., ... Bierut, L.J. (2018). Collaborative meta-analysis finds no evidence of a strong interaction between stress and 5-HTTLPR genotype contributing to the development of depression. *Mol Psychiatry, 23*(1), 133–142. doi: 10.1038/mp.2017.44

Dallos, R., & Johnstone, L. (2014). *Formulation in psychology and psychotherapy*. East Sussex: Routledge.

Daniel, T., & Mcleod, J. (2006). Weighing up the evidence: A qualitative analysis of how person-centred counsellors evaluate the effectiveness of their practice. *Counselling and Psychotherapy Research, 6*(4), 244–249.

Davidson, J., & Bifulco, A. (2018). *Child abuse and protection: Contemporary issues in research, policy and practice*. London: Routledge.

De Bellis, M.D., Baum, A.S., Birmaher, B., Keshavan, M.S., Eccard, C.H., Boring, A.M., ... Ryan, N.D. (1999). Developmental traumatology. Part I: Biological stress systems. *Biological Psychiatry*, *45*(10), 1259–1270.

de Mello, M.F., de Jesus Mari, J., Bacaltchuk, J., Verdeli, H., & Neugebauer, R. (2005). A systematic review of research findings on the efficacy of interpersonal therapy for depressive disorders. *European Archives of Psychiatry and Clinical Neuroscience*, *255*(2), 75–82.

de Shazer, S., Berg, I.K., Lipchik, E., Nunnally, E., Molnar, A., Gingerich, W., & Weiner-Davis, M. (1986). Brief therapy: Focused solution development. *Family Process*, *25*(2), 207–221.

Dean, J., & Goodlad, R. (1998). *Supporting community participation: The role and impact of befriending.* Brighton: Pavilion Publishing/Joseph Rowntree Foundation.

Deaux, K. (1993). Reconstructing social identity. *Personality and Social Psychology Bulletin*, *19*, 4–12. doi: 10.1177/0146167293191001

Department of Work and Pensions. (2015). *Households below average income: 1994/1995 to 2013/2014.* Retrieved from https://www.gov.uk/government/statistics/households-below-average-income-199495-to-201516

Diamond, G.M., Shahar, B., Sabo, D., & Tsvieli, N. (2016). Attachment-based family therapy and emotion-focused therapy for unresolved anger: The role of productive emotional processing. *Psychotherapy*, *53*(1), 34.

Dijkstra, A. (2005). Working mechanisms of computer-tailored health education: Evidence from smoking cessation. *Health Education Research*, *20*(5), 527–539.

Dixon, A.K., Fisch, H.U., Huber, C., & Walser, A. (1989). Ethological studies in animals and man: Their use of psychiatry. *Pharmacopsychiatry*, *22*, 44–50. doi: 10.1055/s-2007–1014624

Dixon, W.A., & Reid, J.K. (2011). Positive life events as a moderator of stress-related depressive symptoms. *Journal of Counseling & Development*, *78*(3), 343–347. doi: 10.1002/j.1556-6676.2000.tb01916.x

Dohrenwend, B.P. (2006). Inventorying stressful life events as risk factors for psychopathology: Toward resolution of the problem of intracategory variability. *Psychol Bull*, *132*(3), 477–449. doi: 10.1037/0033–2909.132.3.477

Dohrenwend, B.S., Askenasy, A.R., Krasnoff, L., & Dohrenwend, B.P. (1978). Exemplification of a method for scaling life events: The PERI life events scale. *Journal of Health and Social Behavior*, *19*(2) 205–229.

Doidge, J.C., Higgins, D.J., Delfabbro, P., Edwards, B., Vassallo, S., Toumbourou, J.W., & Segal, L. (2017). Economic predictors of child maltreatment in an Australian population-based birth cohort. *Children and Youth Services Review*, *72*, 14–25. doi: 10.1016/j.childyouth.2016.10.012

Dong, M., Giles, W.H., Felitti, V.J., Dube, S.R., Williams, J.E., Chapman, D.P., & Anda, R.F. (2004). Insights into causal pathways for ischemic heart disease: Adverse childhood experiences study. *Circulation*, *110*(13), 1761–1766. doi: 10.1161/01.CIR.0000143074.54995.7F

Donoghue, H.M., Traviss-Turner, G.D., House, A.O., Lewis, H., & Gilbody, S. (2016). Life adversity in depressed and non-depressed older adults: A crosssectional comparison of the brief LTE-Q questionnaire and life events and difficulties interview as part of the CASPER study. *Journal of Affective Disorders*, *193*, 31–38. doi: 10.1016/j.jad.2015.12.070

Dozier, M. (2003). Attachment-based treatment for vulnerable children. *Attachment and Human Development*, *5*(3), 253–257.

Dozier, M., Albus, K., Fisher, P.A., & Sepulveda, S. (2002). Interventions for foster parents: Implications for developmental theory. *Development and Psychopathology*, *14*, 843–860.

Drake, B., & Jonson-Reid, M. (2014). Poverty and child maltreatment. In J.E. Korbin & R.D. Krugman (Eds.), *Handbook of child maltreatment* (pp. 131–148). Dordrecht: Springer.

Drasch, K., & Matthes, B. (2013). Improving retrospective life course data by combining modularized self-reports and event history calendars: Experiences from a large scale survey. *Quality & Quantity, 47*(2), 817–838.

Dube, S.R., Anda, R.F., Felitti, V.J., Croft, J.B., Edwards, V.J., & Giles, W.H. (2001). Growing up with parental alcohol abuse: Exposure to childhood abuse, neglect, and household dysfunction. *Child Abuse & Neglect, 25*(12), 1627–1640. doi: 10.1016/S0145-2134(01)00293-9

Dudley, R., & Kuyken, W. (2006). Formulation in cognitive-behavioural therapy:'There is nothing either good or bad, but thinking makes it so'. In D.A. Lane & S. Corrie (Eds.), *Formulation in psychology and psychotherapy* (pp. 34–63). London: Routledge.

Duncan, G.J., Kalil, A., & Ziol-Guest, K.M. (2013). Early childhood poverty and adult achievement, employment and health. *Family Matters, 93*, 27–35.

Eales, M. (1988). Depression and anxiety in unemployed men. *Psychological Medicine, 18*(4) 935–945. doi: 10.1017/S0033291700009867

Elliot, A.J., & Hulleman, C.S. (2017). Achievement goals. *Handbook of competence and motivation: Theory and application, 2*, 43–60.

Ennis, N., Sijercic, I., & Monson, C.M. (2018). Internet-delivered early interventions for individuals exposed to traumatic events: Systematic review. *Journal of Medical Internet Research, 20*(11), e280.

Erwin, B.A., Heimberg, R.G., Marx, B.P., & Franklin, M.E. (2006). Traumatic and socially stressful life events among persons with social anxiety disorder. *Journal of Anxiety Disorders, 20*(7), 896–914. doi: 10.1016/j.janxdis.2005.05.006

Fagundes, C.P., Glaser, R., Johnson, S.L., Andridge, R.R., Yang, E.V., Di Gregorio, M.P., … Bechtel, M.A. (2012). Basal cell carcinoma: Stressful life events and the tumor environment. *Archives of General Psychiatry, 69*(6), 618–626.

Farmer, A., & McGuffin, P. (2003). Humiliation, loss and other types of life events and difficulties: A comparison of depressed subjects, healthy controls and their siblings. *Psychological Medicine, 33*(7), 1169–1175. doi: 10.1017/S0033291703008419

Fearon, P., Target, M., Sargent, J., Williams, L.L., McGregor, J., Bleiberg, E., & Fonagy, P. (2006). Short-term mentalization and relational therapy (SMART): An integrative family therapy for children and adolescents. In J.G. Allen, & P. Fonagy (Eds.), *Handbook of mentalization-based treatment* (pp. 201–222). Toronto: John Wiley & Sons.

Felitti, V.J. (2002). The relationship of adverse childhood experiences to adult health: Turning gold into lead. *Permanente Journal, 6*(1), 44–47.

Felitti, V.J., Anda, R.F., Nordenberg, D., Williamson, D.F., Spitz, A.M., Edwards, V., … Marks, J.S. (1998). Relationship of childhood abuse and household dysfunction to many of the leading causes of death in adults: The adverse childhood experiences (ACE) study. *American Journal of Preventive Medicine, 14*(4), 245. doi: 10.1016/S0749-3797(98)00017-8

Fergusson, D.M., Boden, J.M., & Horwood, J.L. (2008). Exposure to childhood sexual and physical abuse and adjustment in early adulthood. *Child Abuse & Neglect, 32*, 607–619.

Finlay-Jones, R., & Brown, G. (1981). Types of stressful life event and the onset of anxiety and depressive disorders. *Psychological Medicine, 11*(4), 803–815. doi: 10.1017/S0033291700041301

First, M., Gibbon, M., Spitzer, R., & Williams, J. (1996). *Users guide for SCID.* New York: Biometrics Research Dept.

Fisher, H.L., Cohen-Woods, S., Hosang, G.M., Korszun, A., Owen, M., Craddock, N., ... Uher, R. (2013). Interaction between specific forms of childhood maltreatment and the serotonin transporter gene (5-HTT) in recurrent depressive disorder. *Journal of Affective Disorders, 145*(1), 136–141. doi: 10.1016/j.jad.2012.05.032

Fisher, H.L., Cohen-Woods, S., Hosang, G.M., Uher, R., Powell-Smith, G., Keers, R., ... McGuffin, P. (2012). Stressful life events and the serotonin transporter gene (5-HTT) in recurrent clinical depression. *Journal of Affective Disorders, 136*(1–2), 189–193. doi: 10.1016/j.jad.2011.09.016.

Fisher, P.A., Stoolmiller, M., Gunnar, M.R., & Burraston, B.O. (2007). Effects of a therapuetic intervention for foster preschoolers on diurnal cortisol activity. *Psychoneuroendocrinology, 32*, 892–905.

Fjeldheim, C.B., Nöthling, J., Pretorius, K., Basson, M., Ganasen, K., Heneke, R., ... Seedat, S. (2014). Trauma exposure, posttraumatic stress disorder and the effect of explanatory variables in paramedic trainees. *BMC Emergency Medicine, 14*(1), 11. doi: 10.1186/1471-227X-14-11

Foley, D., Neale, M., & Kendler, K. (1996). A longitudinal study of stressful life events assessed at interview with an epidemiological sample of adult twins: The basis of individual variation in event exposure. *Psychological Medicine, 26*(6), 1239–1252.

Fonagy, P., & Target, M. (1997). Attachment and reflective function: Their role in self-organization. *Development and Psychopathology, 9*(4), 679–700.

Forkmann, T., Teismann, T., Stenzel, J.-S., Glaesmer, H., & de Beurs, D. (2018). Defeat and entrapment: more than meets the eye? Applying network analysis to estimate dimensions of highly correlated constructs. *BMC Medical Research Methodology, 18*, 16. doi: 10.1186/s12874-018-0470-5

Fossion, P., Leys, C., Kempenaers, C., Braun, S., Verbanck, P., & Linkowski, P. (2015). Beware of multiple traumas in PTSD assessment: The role of reactivation mechanism in intrusive and hyper-arousal symptoms. *Aging & Mental Health, 19*(3), 258–263. doi: 10.1080/13607863.2014.924901

Freud, S. (1924). Mourning and Melancholia. *The Psychoanalytic Review (1913–1957), 11*(77), 237–258.

Fuhr, K., Reitenbach, I., Kraemer, J., Hautzinger, M., & Meyer, T.D. (2017). Attachment, dysfunctional attitudes, self-esteem, and association to depressive symptoms in patients with mood disorders. *Journal of Affective Disorders, 212*, 110–116. doi: 10.1016/j.jad.2017.01.021

Gaudiano, B.A. (2011). Evaluating acceptance and commitment therapy: An analysis of a recent critique. *International Journal of Behavioral Consultation and Therapy, 7*(1), 54–65. doi: 10.1037/h0100927

Gentzler, A.L., & Kerns, K.A. (2006). Adult attachment and memory of emotional reactions to negative and positive events. *Cognition and Emotion, 20*, 20–42. doi: 10.1080/02699930500200407

Gentzler, A.L., Kerns, K.A., & Keener, E. (2010). Emotional reactions and regulatory responses to negative and positive events: Associations with attachment and gender. *Motivation and Emotion, 34*(1), 78–92. doi: 10.1007/s11031-009-9149-x

Gentzler, A.L., Ramsey, M.A., Yi, C.Y., Palmer, C.A., & Morey, J.N. (2014). Young adolescents' emotional and regulatory responses to positive life events: Investigating temperament, attachment, and event characteristics. *The Journal of Positive Psychology, 92*(2), 108–121. doi: 10.1080/17439760.2013.848374

George, C., Kaplan, N., & Main, M. (1984). *Attachment Interview for Adults*. Berkeley: University of California.

Germine, L., Nakayama, K., Duchaine, B.C., Chabris, C.F., Chatterjee, G., & Wilmer, J.B. (2012). Is the web as good as the lab? Comparable performance from web and lab in cognitive/perceptual experiments. *Psychonomic Bulletin & Review, 19*(5), 847–857.

Gianonne, F., Schimenti, A., Caretti, V., Chiarenza, A., Ferraro, A., Guarino, S., ... Bifulco, A. (2011). Validita attendibilita e proprieta pscyhometriche dela verdsione Italiana dell'intervista CECA (Childhood experience of care and abuse). *Psiciatria e Psicoterapia, 30*, 3–21.

Gibbard, I., & Hanley, T. (2008). A five-year evaluation of the effectiveness of person-centred counselling in routine clinical practice in primary care. *Counselling and Psychotherapy Research, 8*(4), 215–222.

Gilbert, P. (2000). The relationship of shame, social anxiety and depression: The role of the evaluation of social rank. *Clinical Psychology and Psychotherapy, 7*(3), 174–189. doi: 10.1002/1099–0879(200007)7:3<174::AID-CPP236>3.0.CO;2-U

Gilbert, P. (2006). *Stumbling on happiness.* New York: Knopf.

Gilbert, P., & Allan, S. (1998). The role of defeat and entrapment (arrested flight) in depression: An exploration of an evolutionary view. *Psychological Medicine, 28*(3), 585–598. doi: 10.1017/S0033291798006710

Girgus, J.S., & Yang, K. (2015). Gender and depression. *Current Opinion in Psychology, 4*, 53–60. doi: 10.1016/j.copsyc.2015.01.019

Gold, S.D., Marx, B.P., Soler-Baillo, J.M., & Sloan, D.M. (2005). Is life stress more traumatic than traumatic stress? *Journal of Anxiety Disorders, 19*(6), 687–698. doi: 10.1016/j.janxdis.2004.06.002

Gomez, V., Krings, F., Bangerter, A., & Grob, A. (2009). The influence of personality and life events on subjective well-being from a life span perspective. *Journal of Research in Personality, 43*(3), 345–354. doi: 10.1016/j.jrp.2008.12.014

Goodman, R. (1999). The extended version of the strengths and difficulties questionnaire as a guide to child psychiatric caseness and consequent burden. *Journal of Child Psychology and Psychiatry and Allied Disciplines, 40*(5), 791–799.

Goodman, R., Ford, T., Richards, H., Gatward, R. (2000). The development and well-being assessment: Description and initial validation of an integrated assessment of child and adolescent psychopathology. *Journal of Child Psychology and Psychiatry and Allied Disciplines, 41*(5), 645–655.

Goodman, R., Ford, T., Simmons, H., Gatward, R., & Meltzer, H. (2000). Using the strengths and difficulties questionnaire (SDQ) to screen for child psychiatric disorders in a community sample. *British Journal of Psychiatry, 177*, 534–539. doi: 10.1192/bjp.177.6.534

Goodyer, I.M. (1995). Life events and difficulties: Their nature and effects. In I.M. Goodyer (Ed.), *The depressed child and adolescent: Developmental and clinical perspectives* (pp. 171–193). Cambridge: Cambridge university Press.

Gorman, D.M., & Brown, G.W. (1992). Recent developments in life-event research and their relevance for the study of addictions. *British Journal of Addiction, 87*, 837–849.

Gosling, S.D., Vazire, S., Srivastava, S., & John, O.P. (2004). Should we trust web-based studies? A comparative analysis of six preconceptions about internet questionnaires. *American Psychologist, 59*(2), 93.

Gottman, J.M., & Levenson, R.W. (1992). Marital processes predictive of later dissolution: Behavior, physiology, and health. *Journal of personality and social psychology, 63*(2), 221–233.

Gray, S.W., & Wilker, H. (2008). Another look at bereavement groups in rural communities: Using solution-focussed brief therapy to foster resiliency. *Grief Matters: The Australian Journal of Grief and Bereavement, 11*(3), 88.

Griffiths, A.W., Wood, A.M., Maltby, J., Taylor, P.J., & Tai, S. (2014). The prospective role of defeat and entrapment in depression and anxiety: A 12-month longitudinal study. *Psychiatry Research, 216*, 52–59. doi: 10.1016/j.psychres.2014.01.037

Grubaugh, A.L., Long, M.E., Elhai, J.D., Frueh, B.C., & Magruder, K.M. (2010). An examination of the construct validity of posttraumatic stress disorder with veterans using a revised criterion set. *Behaviour Research and Therapy, 48*(9), 909–914. doi: 10.1016/j.brat.2010.05.019

Guðmundsdóttir, K. (2016). *The impact of social trauma among outpatients with social anxiety disorder compared to individuals with no mental disorders.* Retrieved from http://hdl.handle.net/1946/24843

Gunnar, M.R., & Quevedo, K. (2007). The neurobiology of stress and development. *Annual Review of Psychology, 58* 145–173.

Gunnar, M.R., & Vazquez, D.M. (2001). Low cortisol and a flattening of expected daytime rhythm: Potential indices of risk in human development. *Development and psychopathology, 13*(3), 515–538.

Hamel, D., & Pampalon, R. (2002). *Trauma and deprivation in Québec.* Québec: Institut national de santé publique du Québec.

Hammen, C., Ellicott, A., Gitlin, M., & Jamison, K.R. (1989). Sociotropy/autonomy and vulnerability to specific life events in patients with unipolar depression and bipolar disorders. *Journal of Abnormal Psychology, 98*(2), 154.

Hantman, S., & Solomon, Z. (2007). Recurrent trauma: Holocaust survivors cope with aging and cancer. *Social psychiatry and psychiatric epidemiology, 42*(5), 396–402. doi: 10.1007/s00127-007-0177-0

Harkness, K.L., & Monroe, S.M. (2016). The assessment and measurement of adult life stress: Basic premises, operational principles, and design requirements. *Journal of Abnormal Psychology, 125*(5), 727–745. doi: 10.1037/abn0000178

Harkness, K.L., & Wildes, J.E. (2002). Childhood adversity and anxiety versus dysthymia co-morbidity in major depression. *Psychological Medicine, 32*, 1239–1249.

Harris, T. (2006). Volunteer befriending as an intervention for depression: Implications for bereavement care. *Bereavement Care, 25*(2), 27–30.

Harris, T.O., Borsanyi, S., Messari, S., Stanford, K., Cleary, S.E., Shiers, H.M., … Herbert, J. (2000). Morning cortisol as a risk factor for subsequent major depressive disorder in adult women. *British Journal of Psychiatry, 177*, 505–510.

Harris, T., Brown, G.W., & Bifulco, A. (1986). Loss of parent in childhood and adult psychiatric disorder: The role of parental care. *Psychological Medicine, 16*, 641–659. doi: 10.1017/S0033291700010394

Harris, T., Brown, G.W., & Robinson, R. (1999a). Befriending as an intervention for chronic depression among women in an inner city: 1: Randomised controlled trial. *The British Journal of Psychiatry, 174*(3), 219–224.

Harris, T., Brown, G.W., & Robinson, R. (1999b). Befriending as an intervention for chronic depression among women in an inner city: 2: Role of fresh-start experiences and baseline psychosocial factors in remission from depression. *The British Journal of Psychiatry, 174*(3), 225–232.

Harris, T.O., Brown, G.W., & Bifulco, A. (1987). Loss of parent in childhood and adult psychiatric disorder: The role of social class position and premarital pregnancy. *Psychological Medicine, 17*, 163–183.

Harris, T.O., Brown, G.W., & Bifulco, A. (1990). Depression and situational helplessness/mastery in a sample selected to study childhood parental loss. *Journal of Affective Disorders, 20*, 27–41.

Hart, J., Gunnar, M., & Cicchetti, D. (1995). Salivary cortisol in maltreated children: Evidence of relations between neuroendocrine activity and social competence. *Development and psychopathology*, *7*(1), 11–26.

Hartling, L.M., & Luchetta, T. (1999). Humiliation: Assessing the impact of derision, degradation, and debasement. *The Journal of Primary Prevention*, *19*, 259. doi: 10.1023/A:1022622422521

Hasin, D.S., Sarvet, A.L., Meyers, J.L., Saha, T.D., Ruan, W.J., Stohl, M., & Grant, B.F. (2018). Epidemiology of adult DSM-5 major depressive disorder and its specifiers in the United States. *JAMA Psychiatry*, *75*(4), 336–346. doi: 10.1001/jamapsychiatry.2017.4602

Hayes, S., Strosahl, K., & Wilson, K. (1999). *Acceptance and commitment therapy: Understanding and treating human suffering*. New York: Guilford.

Hayes, S.C., Strosahl, K.D., & Wilson, K.G. (2011). *Acceptance and commitment therapy: The process and practice of mindful change*. New York: Guilford Press.

Headey, B. (2006). Subjective well-being: Revisions to dynamic equilibrium theory using national panel data and panel regression methods. *Social Indicators Research*, *79*, 369–403.

Heim, C., Ehlert, U., & Hellhammer, D.H. (2000). The potential role of hypocortisolism in the pathophysiology of stress-related bodily disorders. *Psychoneuroendocrinology*, *25*(1), 1–35.

Heir, T., Blix, I., & Knatten, C.K. (2016). Thinking that one's life was in danger: Perceived life threat in individuals directly or indirectly exposed to terror. *The British Journal of Psychiatry*, *209*(4), 306–310. doi: 10.1192/bjp.bp.115.170167

Helgadóttir, F.D., Menzies, R.G., Onslow, M., Packman, A., & O'Brian, S. (2009). Online CBT I: Bridging the gap between Eliza and modern online CBT treatment packages. *Behaviour Change*, *26*(4), 245–253.

Hiskey, S., & Troop, N.A. (2002). Online longitudinal survey research: Viability and participation. *Social Science Computer Review*, *20*(3), 250–259.

Holmes, T.H., & Rahe, R.H. (1967). The social readjustment rating scale. *Journal of Psychosomatic research*, *11*(2), 213–218. doi: 10.1016/0022–3999(67)90010-4

Horesh, D., Solomon, Z., Zerach, G., & Ein-Dor, T. (2011). Delayed-onset PTSD among war veterans: The role of life events throughout the life cycle. *Social psychiatry and psychiatric epidemiology*, *46*(9), 863–870. doi: 10.1007/s00127-010-0255-6

Hosang, G.M., Fisher, H.L., Cohen-Woods, S., McGuffin, P., & Farmer, A.E. (2017). Stressful life events and catechol-O-methyl-transferase (COMT) gene in bipolar disorder. *Depression and Anxiety*, *34*(5), 419–426.

Hosang, G.M., Korszun, A., Jones, L., Gray, G.M., Gunasinghe, C.M., & Mcguffin, P. (2010). Adverse life event reporting and worst illness episodes in unipolar and bipolar affective disorders: Measuring environmental risk for genetic research. *Psychological Medicine*, *40*(11), 1829–1837. doi: 10.1192/bjp.bp.112.111047

Hosang, G.M., Uher, R., Maugham, B., McGuffin, P., & Farmer, A. (2012). The role of loss and danger events in symptom exacerbation in bipolar disorder. *Journal of Psychiatric Research*, *46*(12), 1584–1589. doi: 10.1016/j.jpsychires.2012.07.009

Huguet, A., Rao, S., McGrath, P.J., Wozney, L., Wheaton, M., Conrod, J., & Rozario, S. (2016). A systematic review of cognitive behavioral therapy and behavioral activation apps for depression. *PLOS ONE*, *11*(5). e0154248. doi: 10.1371/journal.pone.0154248

Hunt, N., Bruce-Jones, W., & Silverstone, T. (1992). Life events and relapse in bipolar affective disorder. *Journal of Affective Disorders*, *25*(1), 13–20.

Hysenbegasi, A., Hass, S.L., & Rowland, C.R. (2005). The impact of depression on the academic productivity of university students. *Journal of mental health policy and economics*, *8*(3), 145.

Ibrahim, A.K., Kelly, S.J., Adams, C.E., & Glazebrook, C. (2013). A systematic review of studies of depression prevalence in university students. *Journal of Psychiatric Research*, *47*(3), 391–400.

Infurna, F.J., Rivers, C.T., Reich, J., & Zautra, A.J. (2015). Childhood trauma and personal mastery: Their influence on emotional reactivity to everyday events in a community sample of middle-aged adults. *PLOS ONE*, *10*(4), e0121840-e0121840. doi: 10.1371/journal.pone.0121840

Infurna, M.R., Reichl, C., Parzer, P., Schimmenti, A., Bifulco, A., & Kaess, M. (2016). Associations between depression and specific childhood experiences of abuse and neglect: A meta-analysis. *Journal of Affective Disorders*, *190*, 47–55. doi: 10.1016/j.jad.2015.09.06

Institute of Medicine. (2015). *Psychosocial interventions for mental and substance use disorders: A framework for establishing evidence-based standards.* Retrieved from Washington, DC. https://www.nap.edu/catalog/19013/psychosocial-interventions-for-mental-and-substance-use-disorders-a-framework

Jacobs, J., & Wolin, S.J. (1989). Alcoholism and family factors: A critical review. In *Galanter, Marc* (Ed), *Recent developments in alcoholism, vol. 7: Treatment research.* (pp. 147–164). New York: Plenum Press.

Jaffee, S.R., Caspi, A., Moffitt, T.E., Polo-Tomás, M., & Taylor, A. (2007). Individual, family, and neighborhood factors distinguish resilient from non-resilient maltreated children: A cumulative stressors model. *Child Abuse & Neglect*, *31*, 231–253.

Jaremka, L.M., Glaser, R., Loving, T.J., Malarkey, W.B., Stowell, J.R., & Kiecolt-Glaser, J.K. (2013). Attachment anxiety is linked to alterations in cortisol production and cellular immunity *Psychological Science*, *24*(3), 272–279. doi: 10.1177/0956797612452571

Jin, Y., Sun, C., Wang, F., An, J., & Xu, J. (2018). The relationship between PTSD, depression and negative life events: Ya'an earthquake three years later. *Psychiatry Research*, *259*, 358–363. doi: 10.1016/j.psychres.2017.09.017

Johansson, R., Ekbladh, S., Hebert, A., Lindström, M., Möller, S., Petitt, E., ... Carlbring, P. (2012). Psychodynamic guided self-help for adult depression through the internet: A randomised controlled trial. *PLOS ONE*, *7*(5) e38021

Johnson, H., & Thompson, A. (2008). The development and maintenance of post-traumatic stress disorder (PTSD) in civilian adult survivors of war trauma and torture: A review. *Clinical Psychology Review*, *28*(1), 36–47. doi: 10.1016/j.cpr.2007.01.017

Johnson, J.G., Han, Y.-S., Douglas, C.J., Johannet, C.M., & Russell, T. (1998). Attributions for positive life events predict recovery from depression among psychiatric inpatients: An investigation of the Needles and Abramson model of recovery from depression. *Journal of Consulting and Clinical Psychology*, *66*(2), 369.

Johnson, S.L., Cuellar, A.K., Ruggero, C., Winett-Perlman, C., Goodnick, P., White, R., & Miller, I. (2008). Life events as predictors of mania and depression in bipolar I disorder: *Journal of Abnormal Psychology*, *117*(2), 268–277. doi: 10.1037/0021-843X.117.2.268

Johnson, S.M. (2003). Introduction to attachment: A therapist's guide to primary relationships and their renewal. In S.M. Johnson & V.E. Whiffen (Eds.), *Attachment processes in couple and family therapy.* London: The Guildford Press.

Joshanloo, M. (2018). Fear and fragility of happiness as mediators of the relationship between insecure attachment and subjective well-being. *Personality and Individual Differences*, *123*, 115–118. doi: 10.1016/j.paid.2017.11.016

Kaess, M., Parzer, P., Mattern, M., Resch, F., Bifulco, A., & Brunner, R. (Jul 2011). Childhood experiences of care and abuse (CECA) – validation of the German version of the questionnaire and interview, and results of an investigation of correlations between adverse childhood experiences and suicidal behaviour. *Zeitschrift fur Kinder- und Jugendpsychiatrie und Psychotherapie, 39*(4), 243–252. doi: 10.1024/1422–4917/a000115

Kaltenthaler, E., Brazier, J., De Nigris, E., Tumur, I., Ferriter, M., Beverley, C., ... Sutcliffe, P. (2006). Computerised cognitive behaviour therapy for depression and anxiety update: A systematic review and economic evaluation. *Health Technology Assessment, 10*(33), 1–168.

Kang, S.-M., Shaver, P.R., Sue, S., Min, K.-H., & Jing, H. (2003). Culture-Specific Patterns in the Prediction of Life Satisfaction: Roles of Emotion, Relationship Quality, and Self-Esteem. *Personality and Social Psychology Bulletin, 29*(12), 1596–1608.

Karg, K., Burmeister, M., Shedden, K., & Sen, S. (2011). The serotonin transporter promoter variant (5-HTTLPR), stress, and depression meta-analysis revisited. *Archives of General Psychiatry, 68*, 444–454. doi: 10.1001/archgenpsychiatry.2010.189

Karlsen, S., Nazroo, J.Y., McKenzie, K., Bhui, K., & Weich, S. (2005). Racism, psychosis and common mental disorder among ethnic minority groups in England. *Psychological Medicine, 35*(12), 1795–1803.

Kazemian, L., Widom, C.S., & Farrington, D.P. (2011). A propsective examination of the relationship between childhood neglect and juvenile delinquency in the Cambridge study in delinquent development. *International Journal of Child, Youth and Family Studies, 1*(2), 65–82.

Kemner, S.M., Mesman, E., Nolen, W.A., Eijckemans, M., & Hillegers, M.H. (2015). The role of life events and psychological factors in the onset of first and recurrent mood episodes in bipolar offspring: Results from the Dutch bipolar offspring study. *Psychological Medicine, 45*(12), 2571–2581.

Kendall, T., Pilling, S., Whittington, C., Pettinari, C., & Burbeck, R. (2005). Clinical Guidelines in Mental Health. II: A guide to making NICE guidelines. *Psychiatric Bulletin, 29*(1), 3–8.

Kendler, K.S., Gatz, M., Gardner, C.O., & Pedersen, N.L. (2006). Personality and major depression: A Swedish longitudinal, population-based twin study. *Archives of General Psychiatry, 63*(10), 1113–1120.

Kendler, K.S., Hettema, J.M., Butera, F., Gardner, C.O., & Prescott, C.A. (2003). Life event dimensions of loss, humiliation, entrapment, and danger in the prediction of onsets of major depression and generalized anxiety. *Archives of General Psychiatry, 60*(8), 789–796. doi: 10.1001/archpsyc.60.8.789

Kendler, K.S., Karkowski, L.M., & Prescott, C.A. (1999). Causal relationship between stressful life events and the onset of major depression. *American Journal of Psychiatry, 156*(6), 837–841.

Kendler, K.S., Kessler, R.C., Walters, E.E., MacLean, C., & et al. (1995). Stressful life events, genetic liability, and onset of an episode of major depression in women. *American Journal of Psychiatry, 152*(6), 833–842.

Kendler, K.S., Neale, M.C., Kessler, R., Heath, A.C., & Eaves, L. (1993). A twin study of recent life events and difficulties. *Archives of General Psychiatry, 50*(10), 789–796. doi: 10.1001/archpsyc.1993.01820220041005

Kendler, K.S., Neale, M.C., Kessler, R.C., Heath, A.C., & Eaves, L.J. (1993). A test of the equal-environment assumption in twin studies of psychiatric illness. *Behavior Genetics, 23*(1), 21–27.

Kendler, K.S., Thornton, L.M., & Prescott, C.A. (2001). Gender differences in the rates of exposure to stressful life events and sensitivity to their depressogenic effects. *American Journal of Psychiatry, 158*(4), 587–593.

Kendler, K.S., Walters, E.E., Neale, M.C., Kessler, R.C., Heath, A., & Eaves, L.J. (1995). The structure of the genetic and environmental risk factors for six major psychiatric disorders in women: Phobia, generalized anxiety disorder, panic disorder, bulimia, major depression, and alcoholism. *Archives of General Psychiatry, 52*(5), 374–383.

Kennedy, E. (2013). Orchids and dandelions: How some children are more susceptible to environmental influences for better or worse and the implications for child development. *Clinical Child Psychology and Psychiatry, 18*(3), 319–321. doi: 10.1177/1359104513490338

Kessler, R.C. (2000). Posttraumatic stress disorder: The burden to the individual and to society. *The Journal of Clinical Psychiatry, 61*(Suppl. 5), 4–14.

Kessler, R.C., Aguilar-Gaxiola, S., Alonso, J., Benjet, C., Bromet, E.J., Cardoso, G., ... Koenen, K.C. (2017). Trauma and PTSD in the WHO World mental health surveys. *European Journal of Psychotraumatology, 8*(Suppl. 5), 1353383. doi: 10.1080/20008198.2017.1353383

Kessler, R.C., Chiu, W.T., Demler, O., Merikangas, K.R., & Walters, E.E. (2005). Prevalence, severity, and comorbidity of 12-month DSM-IV disorders in the national comorbidity survey replication. *Archives of General Psychiatry, 62*(6), 617–627.

Khazanov, G.K., Ruscio, A.M., & Swendsen, J. (2019). The 'brightening effect': Reactions to positive events in the daily lives of individuals with major depressive disorder and generalized anxiety disorder. *Behavior Therapy, 50*(2), 270–284. doi: 10.1016/j.beth.2018.05.008

Kim-Cohen, J., Caspi, A., Taylor, A., Williams, B., Newcombe, R., Craig, I.W., & Moffitt, T.E. (2006). MAOA, maltreatment, and gene-environment interaction predicting children's mental health: New evidence and a meta-analysis. *Molecular Psychiatry, 11*(10), 903–913. doi: 10.1038/sj.mp.4001851

Kim, M.M., Ford, J.D., Howard, D.L., & Bradford, D.W. (2010). Assessing trauma, substance abuse, and mental health in a sample of homeless men. *Health & Social Work, 35*(1), 39–48. doi: 10.1093/hsw/35.1.39

Korszun, A., Moskvina, V., Brewster, S., Craddock, N., Ferrero, F., Gill, M., ... McGuffin, P. (2004). Familiality of symptom dimensions in depression. *Arch Gen Psychiatry, 61*(5), 468–474. doi: 10.1001/archpsyc.61.5.468

Kraines, S.H. (1964). Life stress and mental health: The Midtown Manhattan study. *JAMA, 187*(6), 464. doi: 10.1001/jama.1964.03060190080033

Kupfer, D.J., Frank, E., Perel, J.M., Cornes, C., Mallinger, A.G., Thase, M.E., ... Grochocinski, V.J. (1992). Five-year outcome for maintenance therapies in recurrent depression. *Archives of General Psychiatry, 49*(10), 769–773.

Larsen, S., E., & Berenbaum, H. (2017). Did the DSM-5 improve the traumatic stressor criterion?: Association of DSM-IV and DSM-5 criterion a with posttraumatic stress disorder symptoms. *Psychopathology, 50*(6), 373–378. doi: 10.1159/000481950

Lavy, S., & Littman-Ovadia, H. (2011). All you need is love? Strengths mediate the negative associations between attachment orientations and life satisfaction. *Personality and Individual Differences, 50*(7), 1050–1055. doi: 10.1016/j.paid.2011.01.023

Layard, R. (2006). *The depression report: A new deal for depression and anxiety disorders.* Retrieved from https://www.researchgate.net/publication/4928933_The_Depression_Report_A_New_Deal_for_Depression_and_Anxiety_Disorders

Leary, M.R. (2012). Sociometer theory. In P.A.M. Van Lange, A.W. Kruglanski, & E.T. Higgins (Eds.), *Handbook of theories of social psychology* (pp. 151–159). London: Sage Publications Ltd.

Lee, C., Gavriel, H., Drummond, P., Richards, J., & Greenwald, R. (2002). Treatment of PTSD: Stress inoculation training with prolonged exposure compared to EMDR. *Journal of Clinical Psychology, 58*(9), 1071–1089.

Lee, D.A., Scragg, P., & Turner, S. (2001). The role of shame and guilt in traumatic events: A clinical model of shame-based and guilt-based PTSD. *British Journal of Medical Psychology, 74*(4), 451–466.

Leenstra, A.S., Ormel, J., & Giel, R. (1995). Positive life change and recovery from depression and anxiety: A three-stage longitudinal study of primary care attenders. *The British Journal of Psychiatry, 166*(3), 333–343. doi: 10.1192/bjp.166.3.333

Leserman, J., Drossman, D.A., Li, Z., Toomey, T.C., Nachman, G., & Glogau, L. (1996). Sexual and physical abuse history in gastroenterology practice: How types of abuse impact health status. *Psychosomatic Medicine, 58*(1), 4–15.

LoCascio, M., Infurna, M.R., Guarnaccia, C., Mancuso, L., Bifulco, A., & Giannone, F. (2018). Does childhood psychological abuse contribute to intimate partner violence victimization? An investigation using the childhood experience of care and abuse interview. *Journal of Interpersonal Violence*, ePub: 886260518794512, August 23, 1–27. doi: 10.1177/0886260518794512

Loveday, C. (2016). *The secret world of the brain. What it does, how it works and how it affects behaviour.* London: Andre Deutsch.

Lucas-Thompson, R.G., & Granger, D.A. (2014). Parent–child relationship quality moderates the link between marital conflict and adolescents' physiological responses to social evaluative threat. *Journal of Family Psychology, 28*(4), 538.

Luiselli, J.K., & Fischer, A.J. (2016). *Computer-assisted and web-based innovations in psychology, special education, and health.* San Francisco Academic Press. Elsevier.

Lyketsos, C.G., Nestadt, G., Cwi, J., & Heithoff, K. (1994). The life chart interview: A standardized method to describe the course of psychopathology. *International Journal of Methods in Psychiatric Research. 4*(3), 143–155.

Lyubomirsky, S., & Ross, L. (1999). Changes in attractiveness of elected, rejected, and pre-cluded alternatives: A comparison of happy and unhappy individuals. *Journal of personality and social psychology, 76*, 988–1007. doi: 10.1037/0022–3514.76.6.988

Lyubomirsky, S., & Tucker, K.L. (1998). Implications of individual differences in subjective happiness for perceiving, interpreting, and thinking about life events. *Motivation and Emotion, 22*, 155–186. doi: 10.1037/0022–3514.75.1.166

McCall, G.J., & Simmons, J.L. (1966). *Identities and Interactions.* New York: Free Press

Macaskill, A., & Denovan, A. (2013). Developing autonomous learning in first year university students using perspectives from positive psychology. *Studies in Higher Education, 38*(1), 124–142.

Machell, K., Kashdan, T., Short, J., & Nezlek, J. (2015). Relationships between meaning in life, social and achievement events, and positive and negative affect in daily life. *Journal of Personality, 83*, 287–298. doi: 10.1111/jopy.12103

Main, M., & Cassidy, J. (1988). Categories of response to reunion with the parent at age 6: Predictable from infant attachment classifications and stable over a one-monh period. *Developmental Psychology, 24*(3), 415–426.

Main, M., Kaplan, N., & Cassidy, J. (1985). Security in infancy, childhood and adulthood: A move to the level of representation. In I. Bretherton & E. Waters (Eds.), *Growing points of attachment theory and research.* Chicago, IL: University of Chicago.

Main, M., & Solomon, J. (1986). Discovery of an insecure-disorganized/disoriented attachment pattern. In T.B. Brazelton & M.W. Yogman (Eds.), *Affective development in infancy* (pp. 95–124). Norwood, NJ: Ablex.

Mann, M.M., Hosman, C.M., Schaalma, H.P., & De Vries, N.K. (2004). Self-esteem in a broad-spectrum approach for mental health promotion. *Health Education Research, 19*(4), 357–372.

Marmot, M. (2020). Health equity in England: The Marmot review 10 years on. *The BMJ*. doi: 10.1136/bmj.m693

Marmot, M.G., Shipley, M.J., & Rose, G. (1984). Inequalities in death—specific explanations of a general pattern? *The Lancet, 323*(8384), 1003–1006.

Maslow, A.H. (1971). *The farther reaches of human nature*. New York: Arkana/Penguin Books.

Maunder, R.G. (2009). Assessing patterns of adult attachment in medical patients. *General Hospital Psychiatry, 31*, 123–130.

McCrory, E., De Brito, S., & Viding, E. (2010). Research review: The neurobiology and genetics of maltreatment and adversity. *Journal of Child Psychology and Psychiatry, 5*(10), 1079–1095.

McCrory, E.J., De Brito, S., & Viding, E. (2012). The link between child abuse and psychopathology: A review of neurobiological and genetic research. *Journal of the Royal Society of Medecine, 105*(4), 151–156 doi: 10.1258/jrsm.2011.110222

McCrory, E.J., Gerin, M.I., & Viding, E. (2017). Childhood maltreatment, latent vulnerability and the shift to preventative psychiatry – the contribution of functional brain imaging. *Journal of Child Psychology Psychiatry, 58*(4), 338–357. doi: 10.1111/jcpp.12713.

McCullough, G., Huebner, E.S., & Laughlin, J.E. (2000). Life events, self-concept, and adolescents' positive subjective well-being. *Psychology in the Schools, 37*, 281–290. doi: 10.1002/(SICI)1520–6807(200005)37:3<281::AID-PITS8>3.0.CO;2-2

McKenna, K., Joinson, A.N., Reips, U.-D., & Postmes, T. (2007). *Oxford handbook of internet psychology*. Oxford: Oxford University Press.

McQuaid, J.R., Monroe, S.M., Roberts, J.E., Kupfer, D.J., & Frank, E. (2000). A comparison of two life stress assessment approaches: prospective prediction of treatment outcome in recurrent depression. *Journal of Abnormal Psychology, 109*(4), 787. doi: 10.1037/0021–843X.109.4.787

McQuaid, J.R., Monroe, S.M., Roberts, J.R., Johnson, S.L., Garamoni, G.L., Kupfer, D.J., & Frank, E. (1992). Toward the standardization of life stress assessment: Definitional discrepancies and inconsistencies in methods. *Stress Medicine, 8*(1), 47–56.

Mead, N., Lester, H., Chew-Graham, C., Gask, L., & Bower, P. (2010). Effects of befriending on depressive symptoms and distress: Systematic review and meta-analysis. *The British Journal of Psychiatry, 196*(2), 96–101.

Meinlschmidt, G., & Heim, C. (2005). Decreased cortisol awakening response after early loss experience. *Psychoneuroendocrinology, 30*(6), 568–576.

Meyer, A. (1994). A short sketch of the problems of psychiatry. 1897. *American Journal of Psychiatry, 151*(6), 42–47.

Mikulincer, M. (1998). Attachment working models and the sense of trust: An exploration of interaction goals and affect regulation. *Journal of Personality and Social Psychology, 74*, 1209–1224. doi: 10.1037/0022–3514.74.5.1209

Mikulincer, M., Gillath, O., & Shaver, P.R. (2002). Activation of the attachment system in adulthood: Threat-related primes increase the accessibility of mental representations of attachment figures. *Journal of Personality and Social Psychology, 83*, 881–895.

Millar, J. (2007). Social exclusion and social policy research: Defining exclusion. In D. Abrams, D. Christian, & D. Gordon (Eds.), *Multidisciplinary handbook of social exclusion research*, 1–16. Chichester: Wiley.

Mollica, R.F., McInnes, K., Pool, C., & Tor, S. (1998). Dose-effect relationships of trauma to symptoms of depression and post-traumatic stress disorder among Cambodian survivors of mass violence. *The British Journal of Psychiatry, 173*(6), 482–488. doi: 10.1192/bjp.173.6.482

Monroe, S.M., & Reid, M. (2008). Gene-environment interactions in depression research: Genetic polymorphisms and life-stress procedures. *Psychological Science, 19*(10), 947–956.

Monroe, S.M., Rohde, P., Seeley, J.R., & Lewinsohn, P.M. (1999). Life events and depression in adolescence: Relationship loss as a prospective risk factor for first onset of major depressive disorder. *Journal of Abnormal Psychology, 108*(4), 606–614.

Monroe, S.M., Slavich, G.M., Torres, L.D., & Gotlib, I.H. (2007). Severe life events predict specific patterns of change in cognitive biases in major depression. *Psychological Medicine, 37*(6), 863–871.

Mooy, J.M., De Vries, H., Grootenhuis, P.A., Bouter, L.M., & Heine, R.J. (2000). Major stressful life events in relation to prevalence of undetected type 2 diabetes: The Hoorn study. *Diabetes Care, 23*(2), 197–201.

Moran, P.M., Bifulco, A., Ball, C., & Campbell, C. (2001). Predicting onset of depression: The vulnerability to depression questionnaire. *British Journal of Clinical Psychology, 40,* 411–427.

Murray-Parkes, C. (1985). Bereavement. *British Journal of Psychiatry, 146,* 11–17. doi: 10.1192/bjp.146.1.11

Murray-Parkes, C. (1988). Bereavement as a psychosocial transition: Processes of adaptation to change. *Journal of Social Issues, 44,* 53–65. doi: 10.1111/j.1540–4560.1988.tb02076.x

Musiat, P., Hoffmann, L., & Schmidt, U. (2012). Personalised computerised feedback in E-mental health. *Journal of Mental Health 21*(4), 346–354. doi: 10.3109/09638237.2011.648347

Nanni, V., Uher, R., & Danese, A. (2012). Childhood maltreatment predicts unfavourable course of illness and treatment outcome in depression: A metaanalysis. *American Journal of Psychiatry, 169*(2) 141–151. doi: 10.1176/appi.ajp.2011.11020335

National Collaborating Centre for Mental Health (Great Britain), National Institute for Health, Clinical Excellence (Great Britain), British Psychological Society, & Royal College of Psychiatrists. (2011). *Common mental health disorders: identification and pathways to care* (Vol. 123). London: Royal College of Psychiatrists Publications.

Nazroo, J., Edwards, A., & Brown, G. (1997). Gender differences in the onset of depression following a shared life event: A study of couples. *Psychological Medicine, 27,* 9–19. doi: 10.1017/S0033291796004187

Nazroo, J.Y., Edwards, A.C., & Brown, G.W. (1998). Gender differences in the prevalence of depression: Artefact, alternative disorders, biology or roles? *Sociology of Health & Illness, 20*(3), 312–330.

Neeleman, J., Oldehinkel, A., & Ormel, J. (2003). Positive life change and remission of non-psychotic mental illness: A competing outcomes approach. *Journal of Affective Disorders, 76*(1–3), 69–78.

NICE. (2009). *Depression: The treatment and management of depression in adults (update).* Retrieved from London. https://www.nice.org.uk/guidance/indevelopment/gid-cgwave0725

Nielsen, M.B., Tangen, T., Idsoe, T., Matthiesen, S.B., & Magerøy, N. (2015). Post-traumatic stress disorder as a consequence of bullying at work and at school. A literature review and meta-analysis. *Aggression and Violent Behavior, 21,* 17–24. doi: 10.1016/j.avb.2015.01.001

Nolen-Hoeksema, S., Larson, J., & Grayson, C. (1999). Explaining the gender difference in depressive symptoms. *Journal of personality and social psychology, 77*(5), 1061.

Norris, F.H., & Slone, L.B. (2013). Understanding research on the epidemiology of trauma and PTSD. *PTSD Research Quarterly, 24*(2–3), 1–13.

O'Connor, M.F. (2010). PTSD in older bereaved people. *Aging & Mental Health, 14*(6), 670–678.

O'Connor, P., & Brown, G. (1984). Supportive relationships: Fact or fancy? *Journal of Social and Personal Relationships, 1,* 159–175.

O'Connor, W. & Nazroo, J. (2002). *Ethnic differences in the context and experience of psychiatric illness: a qualitative study.* London: Department of Health. Retrieved from https://www. semanticscholar.org/paper/Ethnic-differences-in-the-Context-and-Experience-of-Nazroo/bfa56a8bd1519fbadb59e1de86795b68d3a8f636

Oldehinkel, A.J., Ormel, J., & Neeleman, J. (2000). Predictors of time to remission from depression in primary care patients: Do some people benefit more from positive life change than others? *Journal of Abnormal Psychology, 109*(2), 299.

Oskis, A., Loveday, C., Hucklebridge, F., Thorn, L., & Clow, A. (2010). Anxious attachment style and salivary cortisol dysregulation in healthy female children and adolescents. *The Journal of Child Psychology and Psychiatry, 52*(2), 111–118. doi: 10.1111/j.1469-7610.2010.02296.x

Panagioti, M., Gooding, P., Taylor, P., & Tarrier, N. (2012). Negative self-appraisals and suicidal behavior among trauma victims experiencing PTSD symptoms: The mediating role of defeat and entrapment. *Depression and Anxiety, 29*(3), 187–194. doi: 10.1002/da.21917

Parker, G., Paterson, A., & Hadzi-Pavlovic, D. (2015). Emotional response patterns of depression, grief, sadness and stress to differing life events: A quantitative analysis. *Journal of Affective Disorders, 175,* 229–232. doi: 10.1016/j.jad.2015.01.015

Paykel, E.S. (1997). The interview for recent life events. *Psychological Medicine, 27*(2), 301–310.

Peace, R. (2001). Social exclusion: A concept in need of definition. *Social Policy Journal of New Zealand, 16,* 17–36. doi: 10.1.1.627.6786

Pfeiffer, P.N., Pope, B., Houck, M., Benn-Burton, W., Zivin, K., Ganoczy, D., ... Nelson, C.B. (2020). Effectiveness of peer-supported computer-based CBT for depression among veterans in primary care. *Psychiatric Services.* doi: 10.1176/appi.ps.201900283

Pohar, R., & Argáez, C. (2017). Acceptance and commitment therapy for post-traumatic stress disorder, anxiety, and depression: A review of clinical effectiveness. Ottawa (ON): Canadian Agency for Drugs and Technologies in Health.

Post, R.M. (1992). Transduction of psychosocial stress into the neurobiology of recurrent affective disorder. *The American Journal of Psychiatry. 149*(8), 999–1010. doi: 10.1176/ajp.149.8.999

Price, J., Sloman, L., Gardner, R., Jr., Gilbert, P., & Rohde, P. (1994). The social competition hypothesis of depression. *British Journal of Psychiatry, 164,* 309–315. doi: 10.1192/bjp.164.3.309

Quoidbach, J., Dunn, E.W., Petrides, K.V., & Mikolajczak, M. (2010). Money giveth, money taketh away: The dual effect of wealth on happiness. *Psychological Science, 21*(6), 759–763. doi: 10.1177/0956797610371963

Ramchandani, P., & Stein, A. (2003). The impact of parental psychiatric disorder on children. *British Medical Journal, 327,* 242–243. doi: 10.1136/bmj.327.7409.242

Ramsey, S.R., Thompson, K.L., McKenzie, M., & Rosenbaum, A. (2016). Psychological research in the internet age: The quality of web-based data. *Computers in Human Behavior, 58,* 354–360.

Rappaport, J., & Seidman, E. (2000). *Handbook of community psychology.* New York: Springer Science & Business Media.

Raskin, N.J., & Rogers, C.R. (2005). Person-centered therapy. In: R.J. Corsini & D. Wedding (Eds.), *Current psychotherapies* (pp. 130–165). Stamford: Thomson Brooks/Cole Publishing Co.

Reyes-Rodríguez, M.L., Rivera-Medina, C.L., Cámara-Fuentes, L., Suárez-Torres, A., & Bernal, G. (2013). Depression symptoms and stressful life events among college students in Puerto Rico. *Journal of Affective Disorders, 145*(3), 324–330.

Richman, W.L., Kiesler, S., Weisband, S., & Drasgow, F. (1999). A meta-analytic study of social desirability distortion in computer-administered questionnaires, traditional questionnaires, and interviews. *Journal of Applied Psychology, 84*(5), 754.

Risch, N., Herrell, R., Lehner, T., Liang, K.-Y., Eaves, L., Hoh, J., ... Ries Merikangas, K. (2009). Interaction between the serotonin transporter gene (5-HTTLPR), stressful life events, and risk of depression: A meta-analysis. *JAMA, 301*(23), 2462–2471.

Rochlen, A.B., Zack, J.S., & Speyer, C. (2004). Online therapy: Review of relevant definitions, debates, and current empirical support. *Journal of Clinical Psychology, 60*(3), 269–283.

Rogers, C.R. (1979). The foundations of the person-centered approach. *Education, 100*(2), 98–107.

Romero-Sanchiz, P., Nogueira-Arjona, R., Garcia-Ruiz, A., Luciano, J.V., Campayo, J.G., Gili, M., ... Lopez-Del-Hoyo, Y. (2017). Economic evaluation of a guided and unguided internet-based CBT intervention for major depression: Results from a multicenter, three-armed randomized controlled trial conducted in primary care. *PLOS ONE, 12*(2): e0172741. doi: 10.1371/journal.pone.0172741

Ronalds, C., Creed, F., Stone, K., Webb, S., & Tomenson, B. (1997). Outcome of anxiety and depressive disorders in primary care. *The British Journal of Psychiatry, 171*(5), 427–433.

Ross, C.E. (2000). Neighborhood disadvantage and adult depression. *Journal of Health and Social Behavior, 41*(2) 177–187.

Rothbaum, B.O. (1997). A controlled study of eye movement desensitization and reprocessing in the treatment of posttraumatic stress disordered sexual assault victims. *Bulletin of the Menninger Clinic, 61*, 317–334.

Rothwell, N. (2005). How brief is solution focussed brief therapy? A comparative study. *Clinical Psychology & Psychotherapy: An International Journal of Theory & Practice, 12*(5), 402–405.

Rutter, M. (1972). *Maternal deprivation reassessed.* Harmondsworth: Penguin.

Rutter, M. (1985a). Family and school influences on behavioural development. *Journal of Child Psychology and Psychiatry and Allied Disciplines, 26*(3), 349–368.

Rutter, M. (1985b). Resilience in the face of adversity: Protective factors and resistance to psychiatric disorder. *British Journal of Psychiatry, 147*, 598–611.

Ruwaard, J., Lange, A., Schrieken, B., Dolan, C.V., & Emmelkamp, P. (2012). The effectiveness of online cognitive behavioral treatment in routine clinical practice. *PLOS ONE, 7*(7) e40089.

Schimmenti, A., & Bifulco, A. (2015). Linking lack of care in childhood to anxiety disorders in emerging adulthood: the role of attachment styles. *Child and Adolescent Mental Health, 20*, 41–48. doi: 10.1111/camh.12051

Schmidt, U., & Wykes, T. (2012). E-mental health–a land of unlimited possibilities. *Journal of Mental Health, 21*(4), 327–331. doi: 10.3109/09638237.2012.705930

Schmit, E.L., Schmit, M.K., & Lenz, A.S. (2016). Meta-analysis of solution-focused brief therapy for treating symptoms of internalizing disorders. *Counseling Outcome Research and Evaluation, 7*(1), 21–39.

Schock, K., Böttche, M., Rosner, R., Wenk-Ansohn, M., & Knaevelsrud, C. (2016). Impact of new traumatic or stressful life events on pre-existing PTSD in traumatized refugees: Results of a longitudinal study. *European Journal of Psychotraumatology, 7*(1), 32106.

Seligman, M.E.P. (2011). *Flourish: A visionary new understanding of happiness and well-being.* New York: Free Press.

Shapiro, F. (1991). Eye movement desensitization and reprocessing procedure: From EMD to EMDR: A new treatment model for anxiety and related traumata. *Behavior Therapist, 14*(5), 133–135.

Shapiro, F. (2017). *Eye movement desensitization and reprocessing (EMDR) therapy: Basic principles, protocols, and procedures.* New York: Guilford Publications.

Shapiro, F., & Maxfield, L. (2002). Eye movement desensitization and reprocessing (EMDR): Information processing in the treatment of trauma. *Journal of Clinical Psychology, 58*(8), 933–946.

Sheinbaum, T., Bifulco, A., Ballespí, S., Mitjavila, M., Kwapil, T.R., & Barrantes-Vidal, N. (2015). Interview investigation of insecure attachment styles as mediators between poor childhood care and schizophrenia-spectrum phenomenology. *PLOS ONE, 10*(8), e0135150 doi: 10.1371/journal.pone.0135150

Siddaway, A.P., Taylor, P.J., Wood, A.M., & Schulz, J. (2015). A meta-analysis of perceptions of defeat and entrapment in depression, anxiety problems, posttraumatic stress disorder, and suicidality. *Journal of Affective Disorders, 184*, 149–159. doi: https://doi.org/10.1016/j.jad.2015.05.046

Simhandl, C., Radua, J., König, B., & Amann, B.L. (2015). The prevalence and effect of life events in 222 bipolar I and II patients: A prospective, naturalistic 4 year follow-up study. *Journal of Affective Disorders, 170*, 166–171.

Slavich, G. M, & Shields, G.S. (2018). Assessing lifetime stress exposure using the stress and adversity inventory for adults (Adult STRAIN): An overview and initial validation. *Psychosomatic Medicine, 80*, 17–27. doi: 10.1097/PSY.0000000000000534

Slavich, G.M., Stewart, J.G., Esposito, E.C., Shields, G.S., & Auerbach, R.P. (2019). The stress and adversity inventory for adolescents (Adolescent STRAIN): Associations with mental and physical health, risky behaviors, and psychiatric diagnoses in youth seeking treatment. *Journal of Child Psychology and Psychiatry, 60*(9), 998–1009. doi:0.1111/jcpp.13038

Smith, D., & Rutter, M. (1995). *Time trends in psychosocial disorder of youth.* Chichester: John Wiley & Sons.

Spence, R., Bunn, A., Nunn, S., Hosang, G.M., Kagan, L., Fisher, H.L., … Bifulco, A. (2015). Measuring life events and their association with clinical disorder: A protocol for development of an online approach. *JMIR Research Protocols, 4*(3), e83. doi: 10.2196/resprot.4085

Spence, R., Kagan, L., & Bifulco, A. (2019). A contextual approach to trauma experience: Lessons from life events research. *Psychological Medicine*, 1–5. doi: 10.1017/50033291719000850

Spence, R., Kagan, L., Nunn, S., Rodriguez, D., Fisher, H.L., Hosang, G.M., & Bifulco, A. (in submission). Attachment style moderates the relationship between positive events and subjective wellbeing.

Spence, R., Nunn, S., & Bifulco, A. (2019). The long-term effects of childhood financial hardship mediated by physical abuse, shame, and stigma on depression in women. *Maltrattamento e Abuso all'Infanzia, 21*, 1. doi: 10.3280/MAL2019-001005

Spence, R., Rodriguez-Bailey, D., Kagan, L., Nunn, S., Fisher, H., Hosang, G., … Bifulco, A. (in press). Life events, depression and supportive relationships affect academic achievement in university students. *Journal of American College Health.* doi: 10.1080/07448481.2020.1841776

Sproston, K., & Nazroo, J. (2002). *Ethnic minority psychiatric illness rates in the community (EMPIRIC).* National Centre for Social Research, Department of Epidemiology &

Public Health, Royal Free and University College Medical School. London: Stationery Office.

Stansfeld, S.A., & Marmot, M.G. (1992). Social class and minor psychiatric disorder in British civil servants: A validated screening survey using the general health questionnaire. *Psychological Medicine, 22*(3), 739–749.

Stein, H., Jacobs, N.J., Ferguson, K.S., Allen, J.G., & Fonagy, P. (1998). What do adult attachment scales measure? *Bulletin of the Menninger Clinic., 62*(1), 33–82.

Sturman, E.D., & Mongrain, M. (2006). Entrapment and perceived status in graduate students experiencing a recurrence of major depression. *Canadian Journal of Behavioural Science / Revue canadienne des sciences du comportement, 40*(3), 185–188. doi: 10.1037/0008-400X.40.3.185

Taylor, A.E., & Munafò, M.R. (2016). Triangulating meta-analyses: The example of the serotonin transporter gene, stressful life events and major depression. *BMC psychology, 4*(1), 23.

Taylor, P.J., Gooding, P., Wood, A.M., & Tarrier, N. (2011). The role of defeat and entrapment in depression, anxiety, and suicide. *Psychological Bulletin, 137*, 391–420. doi: 10.1037/a0022935

Taylor, P.J., Gooding, P., Wood, A.M., & Tarrier, N. (2014). The role of defeat and entrapment in depression, anxiety, and suicide. *Psychiatry Research, 216*, 52–59. doi: 10.1016/j.psychres.2014.01.037

Tennant, R., Hiller, L., Fishwick, R., Platt, S., Joseph, S., Weich, S., & Stewart-Brown, S. (2007). The Warwick-Edinburgh mental well-being scale (WEMWBS): Development and UK validation. *Health Qualitative Life Outcomes, 5*, 63. doi: 10.1186/1477-7525-5-63

Trepper, T.S., Dolan, Y., McCollum, E.E., & Nelson, T. (2006). Steve de Shazer and the future of solution-focused therapy. *Journal of Marital and Family Therapy, 32*(2), 133–139.

Uher, R. (2008). The case for gene-environment interactions in psychiatry. *Current Opinion in Psychiatry, 21*(4), 318–321.

Uher, R., & McGuffin, P. (2008). The moderation by the serotonin transporter gene of environmental adversity in the aetiology of mental illness: Review and methodological analysis. *Molecular Psychiatry, 13*(2), 131–146. doi: 10.1038/sj.mp.4002067

Uher, R., & McGuffin, P. (2010). The moderation by the serotonin transporter gene of environmental adversity in the etiology of depression: 2009 update. *Molecular Psychiatry, 15*(1), 18–22.

van den Born-van Zanten, S., Dongelmans, D.A., Dettling-Ihnenfeldt, D., Vink, R., & van der Schaaf, M. (2016). Caregiver strain and posttraumatic stress symptoms of informal caregivers of intensive care unit survivors. *Rehabilitation Psychology, 61*(2), 173. doi: 10.1037/rep0000081

van der Kolk, B. (2005). Developmental trauma disorder. *Psychiatric Annals, 35*(5), 401–408.

van der Kolk, B. (2015). *The body keeps the score: Mind, brain and body in the transformation of trauma.* London: Penguin.

van der Kolk, B.A. (2001). The assessment and treatment of complex PTSD. In R. Yehuda (Ed.), *Traumatic stress* (1–29). Washington DC: American Psychiatric Press.

van der Kolk, B.A., Pelcovitz, D., Roth, S., Mandel, F.S., & et al. (1996). Dissociation, somatization, and affect dysregulation: The complexity of adaption to trauma. *American Journal of Psychiatry, 153*(Suppl), 83–93.

Van Hooff, M., McFarlane, A.C., Baur, J., Abraham, M., & Barnes, D.J. (2009). The stressor criterion-A1 and PTSD: A matter of opinion? *Journal of Anxiety Disorders, 23*(1), 77–86. doi: https://doi.org/10.1016/j.janxdis.2008.04.001

van IJzendoorn, M.H., Bakermans-Kranenburg, M.J., & Ebstein, R.P. (2011). Methylation matters in child development: Toward developmental behavioral epigenetics. *Child development perspectives*, *5*(4), 305–310.

Vandeleur, C.L., Fassassi, S., Castelao, E., Glaus, J., Strippoli, M.F., Lasserre, A.M., … Preisig, M. (2017). Prevalence and correlates of DSM-5 major depressive and related disorders in the community. *Psychiatry Research*, *250*, 50–58. doi: 10.1016/j.psychres.2017.01.060.

Warren, R.P. (2007). *All the King's men*. London: Penguin Modern Classics.

Watts, J. (2016). IAPT and the ideal image. In J. Lees (Ed.), *The future of psychological therapy* (pp. 84–101). London: Routledge.

Weathers, F.W., Blake, D.D., Schnurr, P.P., Kaloupek, D.G., Marx, B.P., & Keane, T.M. (2013). *The life events checklist for DSM-5 (LEC-5). Instrument available from the National Center for PTSD*. Retrieved from www.ptsd.va.gov

Weigold, A., Weigold, I.K., & Russell, E.J. (2013). Examination of the equivalence of self-report survey-based paper-and-pencil and internet data collection methods. *Psychological Methods*, *18*(1), 53.

Weissman, M.M., Gammon, G.D., John, K., Merikangas, K.R., Warner, V., Prusoff, B.A., & Sholomskas, D. (1987). Children of depressed parents: Increased psychopathology and early onset of major depression. *Archives of General Psychiatry*, *44*(10), 847–853.

Widom, C.S., & Ames, M.A. (1994). Criminal consequences of childhood sexual victimization. *Child Abuse and Neglect*, *18*, 303–318.

Wilhelm, K., Mitchell, P.B., Niven, H., Finch, A., Wedgwood, L., Scimone, A., … Schoefield, P.R. (2006). Life events, first depression onset and the serotonin transporter gene. *British Journal of Psychiatry*, *188*, 210–215.

Wing, J.K., Cooper, J.E., & Sartorius, N. (2012). *Measurement and classification of psychiatric symptoms: An instruction manual for the PSE and CATEGO program*. Cambridge: Cambridge University Press.

Wing, S.K. (Ed.). (2007). *Mass observation: Britain in the Second World War*. London: The Folio Society.

Wood, J.V., Heimpel, S.A., Newby-Clark, I.R., & Ross, M. (2005). Snatching defeat from the jaws of victory: Self-esteem differences in the experience and anticipation of success. *Journal of Personality and Social Psychology*, *89*(5), 764.

Wynaden, D., McAllister, M., Tohotoa, J., Al Omari, O., Heslop, K., Duggan, R., … Byrne, L. (2014). The silence of mental health issues within university environments: A quantitative study. *Archives of Psychiatric Nursing*, *28*(5), 339–344.

Xu, J., & Liao, Q. (2011). Prevalence and predictors of posttraumatic growth among adult survivors one year following 2008 Sichuan earthquake. *Journal of Affective Disorders*, *133*(1–2), 274–280. doi: 10.1016/j.jad.2011.03.034

Young, K.C., Machell, K.A., Kashdan, T.B., & Westwater, M.L. (2018). The cascade of positive events: Does exercise on a given day increase the frequency of additional positive events?. *Personality and Individual Differences*, *120*, 299–303. doi: 10.1016/j.paid.2017.03.032

Appendix 1

Bedford Square team projects utilising the LEDS referred to in findings presented

The studies and findings referred to in this book from the Bedford Square team are outlined below. This does not cover all projects undertaken by the team. All those with findings referred to in the text (apart from study 4) were community-based samples, largely London, and many involved women only. The usual procedure was to send out screening through general practice lists to select respondents. Further details of the samples can be found in the papers listed below. The studies were a mix of cross-sectional retrospective and prospective. Most listed here used the LEDS interview together with a clinical interview and the CECA measure of childhood experience and a proximal vulnerability measure.

Clinical interviews involved either the Present State Examination (PSE) or the Structured Clinical Interview for DSM (SCID). The CLEAR study utilised the General Health Questionnaire (GHQ). The Warwick Edinburgh Mental Wellbeing Scale was used in the CLEAR project.

Vulnerability utilises the Self Esteem and Social Support (SESS) interview and Attachment Style Interview (ASI). A questionnaire – the Vulnerable Attachment Style Questionnaire (VASQ) – validated against the interview was used in the CLEAR study. Prior life adversity measured with the Adult Life Phase Interview (ALPHI).

Childhood measured by the Childhood Experience of Care and Abuse (CECA) interview.

Funding: All studies were MRC funded, apart from the CLEAR project which was ESRC funded and the Genetic study which had Welcome funding.

1969–1971 and 1973–1975

1   **Camberwell study:** Random sample of Camberwell general population – 458 females interviewed cross-sectionally. PSE and LEDS.
    Brown, G. W., & Harris, T. (1978). *Social origins of depression – A study of psychiatric disorder in women*. London: Tavistock Publications.

1980–1985

2 **Loss/danger study:** 164 London community women aged 16–40 who were consulting at a general practice in central London. PSE for depression and anxiety, LEDS, including loss and danger ratings.
   Finlay-Jones, R., & Brown, G. (1981). Types of stressful life event and the onset of anxiety and depressive disorders. *Psychological Medicine, 11*(4), 803–815.

3 **Islington study:** Representative sample of Islington working-class mothers – 404 females, prospectively interviewed three times over three years. LEDS and PSE, SESS for vulnerability and CECA for childhood.
   Brown, G. W., Bifulco, A., & Andrews, B. (1990). Self-esteem and depression: III. Aetiological issues. *Social Psychiatry and Psychiatric Epidemiology, 25*, 235–243.

4 **Patient sample:** Prospective study of 127 women aged 18–60 attending psychiatric departments of two North London hospitals. They were seen in most instances after their condition had shown some improvement and were followed up with a second interview two years later. (Sample used in combination with (study 1) for reporting of humiliation and entrapment events. LEDS and PSE.)
   Brown, G. W., Harris, T. O., & Hepworth, C. (1995). Loss, humiliation and entrapment among women developing depression: A patient and non-patient comparison. *Psychological Medicine, 25*, 7–21.

1990–1995

5 **Coping project:** Women screened for vulnerability free of depression followed up to examine new onset of depression – 100 females followed prospectively for their coping over four time points. LEDS, SESS, ASI and CECA. SCID for disorder.
   Bifulco, A., Brown, G. W., Moran, P., Ball, C., & Campbell, C. (1998). Predicting depression in women: The role of past and present vulnerability. *Psychological Medicine, 28*(1), 39–50.

6 **Sisters study:** Women comprising sister pairs, half of whom were selected for the experience of childhood adversity (200 females). CECA, ALPHI, ASI and SCID lifetime disorder.
   Bifulco, A., Bernazzani, O., Moran, P. M., & Ball, C. (2000). Lifetime stressors and recurrent depression: Preliminary findings of the Adult Life Phase Interview (ALPHI). *Social psychiatry and psychiatric epidemiology, 35*, 264–275. doi:10.1007/s001270050238

7 **Couples study:** 100 pairs in Bethnal Green selected by postal screening of the wives for the joint experience of a severe event/major difficulty with their partners. LEDS, PSE and CECA.
   Nazroo, J., Edwards, A., & Brown, G. (1997). Gender differences in the onset of depression following a shared life event: A study of couples. *Psychological Medicine, 27*, 9–19. doi:10.1017/S0033291796004187

8 **Befriending project:** Women with chronic depression tested with a be-friending intervention – 108 females from Islington G.P. lists – followed up after intervention/control group status. LEDS, PSE, SESS and ASI.

Harris, T., Brown, G. W., & Robinson, R. (1999). Befriending as an inter-vention for chronic depression among women in an inner city: 1: Ran-domised controlled trial. *The British Journal of Psychiatry, 174*(3), 219–224.

1995–1998

9 **Cortisol Project:** Islington vulnerable women – 120 females – followed prospectively with baseline measure of salivary cortisol as well as psychoso-cial measures. LEDS, PSE, SESS, ASI and CECA.

Harris, T. O., Borsanyi, S., Messari, S., Stanford, K., Cleary, S. E., Shiers, H. M., … Herbert, J. (2000). Morning cortisol as a risk factor for subse-quent major depressive disorder in adult women. *British Journal of Psy-chiatry, 177*, 505–510.

2006–2009

10 **Genetic study** of community women n = 302: Recontact of 119 Isling-ton women previously studied (studies 3, 4 and 7). Additional Southwark & Oxford samples (Herbert) (n = 183). Measures CECA, LEDS and SESS to-gether with genotyping.

Brown, G. W., Ban, M., Craig, T. K., Harris, T. O., Herbert, J., & Uher, R. (2013). Serotonin transporter length polymorphism, childhood mal-treatment, and chronic depression: a specific gene–environment inter-action. *Depression and Anxiety, 30*(1), 5–13.

2012–2015

11 **CLEAR project:** An online measure of life event – validation using the LEDS. Sample involved recontact of the Depression Case Control sample plus a student group. CLEAR life events, LEDS for validity, GHQ, VASQ and WEWMS.

Bifulco, A., Kagan, L., Spence, R., Nunn, S., Bailey-Rodriquez, D., Hosang, G. M., … Fisher, H. L. (2019). Characteristics of severe life events, at-tachment style and depression - Using an online approach. *The British Journal of Clinical Psychology*, 1–13. doi:10.1111/bjc.1221

Index

Note: **Bold** page numbers refer to tables; *italic* page numbers refer to figures and page numbers followed by "n" denote endnotes.

For Product Safety Concerns and Information please contact our EU
representative GPSR@taylorandfrancis.com
Taylor & Francis Verlag GmbH, Kaufingerstraße 24, 80331 München, Germany